STATEMENT CONCERNING PUBLICATIONS OF
RUSSELL SAGE FOUNDATION

Russell Sage Foundation was established in 1907 by Mrs. Russell Sage "for the improvement of social and living conditions in the United States of America." In carrying out its purpose the Foundation maintains a staff which, among other duties, conducts studies of social conditions, authorized by the General Director, where new information, its analysis and interpretation seem necessary in order to formulate and advance practicable measures aimed at improvement. From time to time the Foundation publishes the results of these studies in book or pamphlet form.

In formulating the problem for study, in mapping out a plan of work on it, in collecting facts, in drawing conclusions, and in the presentation of findings, authors of Foundation studies, who are always either members of the staff or specially commissioned research workers, have the benefit of the criticism and advice of their colleagues in the organization. Full freedom is given research workers for the final decision on all of these steps, and in presenting and interpreting both factual material and conclusions in their own way. While the general responsibility for management of the Foundation is vested in the Board of Trustees, the responsibility for facts, conclusions, and interpretations rests with the research workers alone and not upon the Foundation, its trustees, or other members of the staff. Publication under the imprint of the Foundation does not imply agreement by the organization or its members with opinions or interpretations of authors. It does imply that care has been taken that the research on which a book is based has been thoroughly done.

NURSING FOR THE FUTURE

A REPORT PREPARED FOR THE
NATIONAL NURSING COUNCIL

By

ESTHER LUCILE BROWN, Ph.D.

Director, Department of
Studies in the Professions
RUSSELL SAGE FOUNDATION

"Landmark Study"
SH 2/07

NEW YORK
RUSSELL SAGE FOUNDATION
1948

WM. F. FELL CO., PRINTERS
PHILADELPHIA

CONTENTS

3

PROFESSIONAL ADVISORY COMMITTEE

Chairman: PEARL McIVER, chief, Office of Public Health Nursing, United States Public Health Service, Washington, D. C.

VIRGINIA M. DUNBAR, dean, Cornell University-New York Hospital School of Nursing; director, Nursing Service, New York Hospital

SISTER M. OLIVIA GOWAN (O.S.B.), dean, School of Nursing Education, Catholic University of America, Washington, D. C.

HEIDE L. HENRIKSEN, assistant chief of nursing operations, Federal Employee Health Division, United States Public Health Service, Washington, D. C.

RUTH W. HUBBARD, president, National Organization for Public Health Nursing; general director, Visiting Nurse Society of Philadelphia

ESTELLE MASSEY OSBORNE, formerly consultant, National Nursing Council, Inc.; instructor, Department of Nursing Education, New York University

LUCILE PETRY, chief, Division of Nursing, United States Public Health Service, Washington, D. C.

ELIZABETH K. PORTER, professor of nursing education, University of Pennsylvania, Philadelphia

RUTH SLEEPER, president, National League of Nursing Education; director, Nursing Service and School of Nursing, Massachusetts General Hospital, Boston

DOROTHY WILSON, assistant professor of nursing education, Teachers College, Columbia University, New York

ANNA DRYDEN WOLF, director, School of Nursing and Nursing Service, The Johns Hopkins Hospital, Baltimore

Ex Officio:

MARJORIE B. DAVIS, executive secretary, National Nursing Council, New York

ADELAIDE C. MAYO, executive secretary, National League of Nursing Education, New York

BLANCHE PFEFFERKORN, director of studies, National League of Nursing Education, New York

5

LAY ADVISORY COMMITTEE

Chairman: WILLIAM HARDING JACKSON, president, Board of Governors, The New York Hospital

MRS. AUGUST BELMONT, Board of Directors, American National Red Cross

KENNETH D. BENNE, associate professor of education, Teachers College, Columbia University, New York

MRS. CHESTER BOLTON, House of Representatives, Congress of the United States

A. J. BRUMBAUGH, vice-president, American Council on Education, Washington, D. C.

LAWRENCE K. FRANK, director, Caroline Zachry Institute of Human Development, New York

LUTHER GULICK, president, Institute of Public Administration, New York

MRS. JOSEPH M. HOWORTH, principal attorney, Office of Legislation, Veterans Administration, Washington, D. C.

EARL LOMON KOOS, professor of sociology, University of Rochester

CHARLES A. ROVETTA, dean of students, University of Chicago

MRS. ARTHUR H. SPIEGEL, treasurer, Chicago Council on Community Nursing

BERNHARD J. STERN, lecturer in sociology, Columbia University, New York

MRS. VANDERBILT WEBB, vice-president, Board of Managers, Bellevue Schools of Nursing, New York

INTRODUCTION

FOR a quarter of a century leaders of nursing education have striven with almost unparalleled zeal but with distressingly small results, many of them believe, to create a sound and socially motivated form of nursing education. Long ago they became convinced that a system of apprenticeship, such as existed in the majority of the training schools, then numbering almost two thousand, was no longer adequate to prepare nurses either for the increasingly complex demands of institutional nursing or for that vast new field of community nursing which was in process of development.

Josephine Goldmark's distinguished report, Nursing and Nursing Education in the United States, published in 1923 under the auspices of the Committee for the Study of Nursing Education, concerned itself with the problem of the reorientation of professional practice to meet new health and social goals, and made specific recommendations for education for such reorientation. Three years later the Committee on the Grading of Nursing Schools began its prodigious task, to which nearly ten years and a quarter of a million dollars were devoted, of attempting to eliminate weak nursing schools and to raise appreciably standards in remaining schools.

Concurrently the national professional associations, particularly the National League of Nursing Education and the National Organization for Public Health Nursing, were continuously making smaller specialized studies and were seeking through a wide variety of educational devices to elevate the practice of, and the preparation for, nursing.

Every attempt achieved something of significance. Accomplishment was larger, however, in indicating the direction in which the profession believed movement should proceed than in

7

initiating or accelerating that movement. The several attempts did succeed in closing many very poor training schools; in opening some university or collegiate schools; in persuading many hospitals to substitute graduate staff nurses in considerable numbers for student nurses; in encouraging hospital schools to lengthen and improve their preclinical period of instruction and to provide more and broader clinical instruction.

Even before World War II put tremendous strain upon all our American institutions, it was apparent that these gains were extremely inadequate. The existing system of nursing education was still incompetent to produce the requisite amount of *qualified* general nursing care needed by expanding health services. It was even more incompetent to produce anything like the required supply of nurses with necessary preparation for such essential functions as specialized clinical nursing, public health nursing, supervision, planning and administration, research and writing.

Through the strenuous exertions of bodies like the National Nursing Council for War Service,[1] American Hospital Association, American Medical Association, and United States Public Health Service with its allocation of funds both to cadet nurses and to schools of nursing, the quantitative supply of nursing care was greatly enlarged during the war years. But no such immediate preparation of large numbers of nursing specialists was possible because specialization requires unhurried time for intellectual and emotional growth, and because most graduate nurses did not have an academic base on which specialization

[1] The National Nursing Council for War Service was created in 1942 from the existent Nursing Council on National Defense for the purpose of coordinating the war efforts of several national organizations. Although established only for the duration of the war, the Council has continued to exist expressly to complete three projected studies, of which this report is one. The constituent bodies are: American Nurses' Association, National League of Nursing Education, National Organization for Public Health Nursing, Association of Collegiate Schools of Nursing, National Association of Colored Graduate Nurses, American Red Cross Nursing Service, Council of Federal Nursing Services, International Council of Nurses, Division of Nursing of U. S. Public Health Service, American Hospital Association, National Association for Practical Nurse Education, American Medical Association, Nursing Unit of U. S. Children's Bureau, American Association of Industrial Nurses.

might be built. Although several thousand registered nurses availed themselves of federal or other scholarships for limited periods of study, the training received was of an emergency nature and more nearly comparable to short-term postgraduate work than true preparation for a specialty.

Many nurses of large potential ability acquired competence, to be sure, in supervision, planning, administration, and teaching, through having to meet the exigencies of war positions into which they were thrust, often against their will or better judgment. To swim or to sink was the alternative faced. For every one who learned quickly enough to swim, there were undoubtedly others who sank into frustration and despair. The situation was not psychologically wholesome for thousands of nurses confronted with great responsibility for which they had had little or no preparation and experience. It was positively hazardous for the health services to which society has entrusted its physical, and is increasingly entrusting its emotional, well-being.

The war finally came to an end—so it was supposed. The National Nursing Council ceased to recruit nurses; the United States Public Health Service no longer received funds for distribution in order to attract young women to nursing. The "nurse's aides" who had rendered such indispensable voluntary service to hospitals during the war years returned to their pleasant and comfortable homes. Soon it was discovered, however, that the war emergency had ended for institutional and community health agencies even less than for the world at large. Patients continued to pour into hospitals and health clinics. With or without money in their pockets, they came to claim the health care that a long continuing program of education had led them to demand. In this they were aided by society as a whole, which visualized greatly enlarged and better distributed health service, readily available to the total population, as the promise of postwar America. The Congress, state legislatures, city councils, community chests and hospital funds, prepayment plans, groups

9

of private citizens, and individual philanthropists had already begun to vote, obtain, or contribute hard, cold cash to make these services a reality.

In many a hospital, however, entire wards or even floors still remained closed because there were not enough nurses to permit reopening. Persons charged with administrative functions grew increasingly alarmed about how whole new institutions were to be staffed. Throughout the nation health agencies had made budgetary provision for positions for which they could find no suitable personnel. Some agencies, in fact, were asked to sacrifice public health nurses to care for the ill in hospitals. Thus the inherent promise of help to the public in preventing disease and *maintaining health* was being jeopardized in order that persons who had not maintained health might receive institutional therapy. The situation everywhere was exceptionally critical in connection with the recruiting of those specialists upon whom the success or failure of any nursing service so largely depends. There were actually hundreds of positions carrying maximum salary and prestige in the supervisory, planning, administrative, and teaching categories, either unfilled or still filled by persons of inadequate ability and preparation.

The nursing profession again concluded that there was something not only drastically but chronically wrong with a system of education which could not meet the demand either for qualitative or quantitative service. Once more it decided to commission the making of a study, in the hope that impetus might be provided for the redirection of effort. This time it was the National Nursing Council that took the initiative by requesting financial support from the Carnegie Corporation of New York for an examination of the question of who should organize, administer, and finance *professional* schools of nursing.

The Council realized that attention was thus being focused on only one portion of the problem. It would have liked to embark on a comprehensive survey of preparation for all nursing functions and not merely of education on the more advanced levels. Such surveys, however, are long, difficult, and expensive. Hence the Council decided to concentrate upon a segment of the total problem. It thought the probability great, moreover, that any answer to the designated question might illuminate related questions.

Subsequently the National Nursing Council asked the writer to serve as director of the study. In an exploratory conference the Council suggested that the director be provided with a Professional Advisory Committee, whose counsel she might seek as needed but which should serve only in a consultative capacity. Because of the large stake that American society has in nursing, it was proposed that there be also a Lay Advisory Committee, representative of the public interest. Later, as the study advanced, a group of hospital administrators and physicians, charged by various organizations with planning for future nursing services, was asked to share in the consideration of the evolving report.

During the preliminary discussions three basic decisions were agreed upon. First, and most important, was the decision to view nursing service and nursing education in terms of what is best for society—not what is best for the profession of nursing as a possibly "vested interest." If it was found that the larger interests of society conflicted at any point with the interests of nurses, the director would be expected to represent the social welfare. This position seemed imperative were the American public to be offered any convincing statement that serious effort had been made to view a difficult and emotionally explosive subject with such unbiased objectivity as was possible.

Second, it was decided that the director should make as extended a field trip through the United States as time permitted. It was thought inexpedient, if not actually dangerous, for observation to be confined to the New York metropolitan area or even to the eastern seaboard, neither of which is typical of the nation. The United States is a vast, sprawling country, rich in the diversity of its geography and economy; its racial, ethnic, and religious groups; its ways of viewing the task of living. Within its borders flourish many scores of regional adaptations to specific conditions and needs. For the very reason that they are adaptations, they often have a validity and a vitality far greater than would any programs, however carefully devised, that were imposed from outside. Hence it was deemed requisite that visits be made at least to some of these experimental laboratories where diversified change is in process of being tested.

The third decision was the outgrowth of discussion about how an answer might be found to the question of who should organize, administer, and finance professional schools of nursing. There appeared but one way to arrive at an answer which could even purport to be sound, and that was by a long, circuitous route. First, as clear a picture as possible would have to be drawn of the probable nature of health services in the second half of the twentieth century, and of the nursing services likely to be demanded by those evolving health services. Next, inquiry into the kinds of training and of academic and professional education requisite to prepare nurses to render those various kinds of nursing services would be essential. Only after these tasks had been completed, could one wisely examine the specific question to which the National Nursing Council was directing attention.

There seemed to be possible usefulness in this circuitous approach for another reason. The Council had asked for a study primarily concerned with basic preparation for specialized nursing services, including specialized clinical nursing. But at a moment when the supply merely of "hands and feet" to perform nursing duties was so precariously low, the health services and the public found it difficult to think of other than a quantitative supply. The need for hands and feet understandably came first in their minds. Interest in a report the chief focus of which was upon greater competence for the truly professional areas of nursing would probably be negligible unless they could see that there was also sincere concern about *their* problem. If it could so much as be indicated—through a discussion of nursing services and training and education for several kinds of such services— that some alleviation of the quantitative problem was possible, their sympathetic understanding and needed support might perhaps be rallied.

These three major decisions were reached with the complete accord of the National Nursing Council, the director of the study, and others interested. For all except the Council, consent presented no difficulty. They wished to see readjustments made that would serve the social interest, as well as the broader interests of the profession of nursing. But for the Council to assent without hesitation was an act little short of greatness. By that act it had signed away "control" of the study. It had given to a member of the laity the right to travel where she would; to consult with physicians, hospital administrators, and others who did not always see eye to eye with nurse administrators and educators; and to prepare a report that might conceivably be at wide variance with the interests of nurses.

The Council was willing to take her and also society on faith. Nursing would benefit over the years, said the representative, in direct proportion to its ability to serve the public welfare. Hence attention ought to be centered on the community at large and its needs, not on nurses. This point of view augurs well for the future of the profession of nursing. Many other professional associations have expressed grave fear over the possibility of "losing control" of studies of themselves. Many have kept their attention so focused upon professional rights and prerogatives that society has sometimes come to question their interest in serving the needs of our national life.

The writer wishes to record that the nursing profession has lived up well to the letter of freedom it initially gave her. As the report nears the end, furthermore, many nurse leaders have expressed satisfaction that the study was undertaken within the broader frame of reference. They have also expressed gratification that it is to be published for general consideration without formulation of majority and minority reports, the usefulness of which is often questionable.

Only once did members of the profession attempt, through other than directly requested means, to influence the report. In that instance an appreciably large and important segment of nursing education had become profoundly disturbed about what it thought the report might include, and the use to which other segments of nursing education might put the recommendations. These representatives of schools were momentarily afraid of change that not only seemed to be imminent, but which they feared would come so rapidly that they could not adjust to it. They met the situation by attending one of the three regional conferences, to which reference will be made later, in unexpectedly large numbers. Their active participation in that conference was, however, of great value. It provided the director with an opportunity to obtain more fully their opinions, to get "the sense of the meeting." The occasion enabled them, she believes, to realize that her report at most would present *a way* of looking at the current situation in nursing education. The profession will be entirely free to use or discard, as it sees fit, the recommendations that are included.

Within a democratic society there is no person, group of persons, or organized voluntary body that has power to order sudden and drastic change. Such changes as are effected will result from long and careful planning at the conference table of national, state, and local nursing associations and other bodies, and of state boards of nurse examiners. More importantly, they will issue from the persistent and courageous efforts of hundreds of nurse educators working within their own schools and communities. The writer is of the opinion that many of those very persons who were most disturbed about possible implications for the future of their schools will be found in the years ahead actively and successfully bringing about change in their institutions.

The fact that the National Nursing Council vested in the director the maximum possible degree of freedom does not indicate that many other persons have not largely participated in the formulation of ideas expressed in the report. Probably over two thousand have had a part in it. For the particular ideas selected from a half-year of conversation with individual persons and groups, for the way in which these ideas have been utilized, and for the conclusions and recommendations drawn from them, the writer must assume complete responsibility. But for the wealth of factual data and opinion, including reports of organizational structure, financing, curriculum construction, instructional methods, and experimental undertakings; provision for the observation of academic and clinical teaching facilities; suggestions for change presented both informally and as written resolutions—for all these contributions that compose the basic source materials underlying the report, credit must go to those some two thousand persons scattered throughout the United States.

A brief résumé of who those persons are and the roles played by them is requisite. The names of the Professional Advisory Committee and the Lay Advisory Committee, to which reference has already been made, appear at the beginning of this report. The interest of the constituency of the Professional Advisory Committee lies primarily in nursing education, whether within the school of nursing or the community nursing agency. All of these women have rendered or are rendering distinguished service in behalf of such education. They were exceptionally helpful during a three-day period at the beginning of the study when they attempted to formulate their opinion of what the implications of the nursing service of the future would be for nursing education.

Several of the members of the Lay Advisory Committee are connected with institutions that engage either in university teaching and research or in the formulation of educational policy. Two of them are authors of studies made expressly for professional nursing associations. Others, not directly associated with educational institutions, have given many years of voluntary service to the encouragement and upbuilding of nursing and nursing education. The chairman, William Harding Jackson, a lawyer by profession, is the president of the Board of Governors of The New York Hospital. In that capacity he had earlier offered strong support in making the School of Nursing, long conducted by The Society of The New York Hospital, a degree-conferring unit of Cornell University.

The third group met formally was composed almost exclusively of physicians and hospital administrators who, officially or unofficially, are particularly interested in the future of nursing and nursing education. Several of them, serving as chairmen or members of committees on nursing or representing organizations such as the American Medical Association and the American Hospital Association, suggested the desirability of conferences at which the general scope and content of the report might be discussed.

A totally different kind of assistance came from the "workshop," which was organized by the executive secretary of the National Nursing Council for the purpose of providing the director with suggestions concerning the probable nature of nursing in the second half of the twentieth century: that question, it will be recalled, that appeared to need an answer before nursing education could profitably be considered. As constituted, the workshop was composed of 19 graduate nurses from scattered parts of the United States who were then engaged in the administration, supervision, or actual practice of nursing service, whether in hospitals, public health and rehabilitation agencies, industry, or private duty. Lawrence K. Frank, director of the Caroline

Zachry Institute of Human Development, was the chairman. He contributed much, as the nurses reported, to their understanding of developmental social factors affecting human welfare, and to the effect which these factors will have upon the professional groups that provide health services.

The extensive memoranda prepared by the workshop during its ten-day session in the spring of 1947 and subsequently, lie before the writer as she sets down this paragraph. The vision of, and insight into, professional nursing at its best—and as the group earnestly hopes it will be practiced in the years ahead—which underscore these materials, provide one of the exceedingly promising indications for the future. Given intellectual leadership such as that inherent in this workshop multiplied a thousand times, and the future of the profession of nursing would be assured. Although reference will be made directly or indirectly to the workshop memoranda, it is regretted that no appreciable part of them can be reproduced in this report.

Different in nature was the help gained from visits to some 50 schools of nursing. These schools were selected for several reasons: variety in regional distribution, organizational structure and control, financing, purpose. Partly by circumstance, more were visited in the South and on the Pacific Coast than in other regions. Some of the schools were operated by hospitals, others by universities, two by a medical school. One was an independent, incorporated "central school." Many of the "hospital schools" had developed an affiliation, of at least a tenuous kind, with an institution of higher learning.

Schools conducted both by voluntary and by public hospitals were seen. A considerable proportion of those in the former category were under sectarian auspices, either Catholic or Protestant. Where they were Catholic, they were operated by religious orders of Sisters. In the latter category were two county hospitals, one municipal and one state hospital, and two federally administered or financed hospitals.

17

Of the five schools on the list that prepared only Negro students, one was under a hospital federally supported, one within a municipal hospital, one within a voluntary hospital. The fourth was conducted by a state university for Negroes; the fifth by a medical school that operated programs for white medical, dental, nursing, and pharmaceutical students, as well as the Negro school of nursing.

In general, effort was made to visit "better" schools in every region. Miserable schools of nursing had been seen at sundry times in various places. No virtue was inherent in further examination of what should not be done. Only schools that attempted to be dynamic and experimental in their approach to nursing education, and that had a reasonably desirable environment within which to work, were likely to provide concept and practice for further development.

These visits afforded an opportunity both to hear and to see. Although the fact that the writer is not a nurse greatly handicapped her ability to observe, walking of numerous hospital wards accompanied by a member of the educational staff and trips to public health agencies used for student field work were exceedingly profitable experiences. The situation in nursing education in the half-hundred schools seemed both better and worse than had been expected. It was better in the imagination and perspective with which nursing education had come to be conceived the country over. Because of totally inadequate financial resources and insufficient numbers of well-prepared teaching personnel, it was disappointingly backward in many places in the extent to which it had been able to translate imagination and perspective into operating educational programs.

Three regional conferences provided still another opportunity for the director to obtain valuable guidance. They were conceived and planned for, as was the workshop, by the executive secretary of the Council. She knew the director of the study could not visit more than a relatively small number of schools. She decided, therefore, to widen the basis of consultation by inviting the directors of the some 1,250 schools of nursing to one of the three-day conferences, in Washington, San Francisco, or Chicago. The director of each school, furthermore, was invited to come accompanied by one other person, who might be an administrative official of her hospital or university, a member of the board of trustees of the hospital or of the nursing committee of the school, or a member of her own administrative or teaching staff. Also invited were representatives of state boards of nurse examiners, federal agencies with nursing units, many official and nonofficial public health agencies, state branches of the National Organization for Public Health Nursing, the American National Red Cross, and two life insurance companies that employ large nursing staffs. Thus it was hoped to obtain opinion from other immediately interested persons besides the directors of schools themselves. Although representatives had to arrange for their own traveling expenses and also a considerable registration fee, more than one thousand persons attended the three conferences.

The conferences were operated primarily as workshops. Each representative was assigned to a particular small group for the entire period of the conference. A list of topics to be discussed by the several groups had been mailed in advance to those invited with the request that they designate first, second, and third choices. So far as possible, assignment was on the basis of designation.

For the purpose of enhancing the productivity both of the general conference sessions and of the work groups, the executive secretary procured the services of teams of university men who have had experience in the relatively new field of "group dynamics." Under the general leadership of Professor Ronald O. Lippitt of the Institute for Research in Group Dynamics of Massachusetts Institute of Technology, Professor Kenneth D. Benne of Columbia University, and Professor Alvin Zander of the University of Michigan, these service teams, together with the executive secretary of the Council and the director of the study, planned and conducted the programs of the general conference sessions. The teams also assumed responsibility for the preliminary training and the guidance of leaders, recorders, and observers who were assigned to the individual groups to aid in their discussions.

At the final session of each conference, the contributions of the several groups were presented, whether in the form of statements, recommendations, or resolutions, to the entire membership, including the director of the study.

If space were available, a detailed statement would be given of the methodology used in the conferences, and of the opinion of the participants concerning the results achieved and the utility of that methodology. Fortunately a report, A Thousand Think Together, constituting the detailed record of both method and content, has been prepared and distributed by the Council to those attending the conferences and others requesting the monograph. It is only possible to note that the writer herself, who participated in the group dynamics process for the first time, is convinced that here is a method, capable of much further expansion and refinement, whereby groups of persons may be helped to think and to act together, and actually to enjoy so doing. She sees in it a constructive instrumentality for achieving democratic thought and action.

At the same time that the representatives of nursing education were struggling to provide the director with the best possible product of group opinion, many of them, she believes, experienced a broadening of their imagination, a greater sense of security through more reliance upon the group rather than upon their individual endeavors, and an insight into the future applicability of some of the methods and concepts to situations "back home." However that may be, members of several other professional groups expressed frank envy that a similar opportunity to participate in a group dynamics conference had not been provided them.

Lest anyone begin to think that the director's consultations were limited largely to administrators of nursing education and their faculties, further note must be made of those members of other health services and of other university personnel who contributed opinion to this study. If there were a medical school in the university whose school of nursing the writer was visiting, an attempt was made to learn about any current developments that had broad implications for nursing education. If plans for the extension of community health care, whether on a private or a public basis, were under local consideration, representatives of those plans were interviewed. Were a university contemplating the creation of a school of nursing or the strengthening and enlargement of its existent school, the president or appropriate dean was consulted. In many places opportunity was provided to confer with hospital administrators. At the regional conferences "resource" persons drawn largely from university faculties and public health agencies were present. In these several ways contacts were made with many physicians and others, a considerable proportion of whom were interested in predicting the future of the health services, and of the profession of nursing whose social function is so closely intertwined with that of medicine.

One professor of preventive medicine was convinced of the way the report should be written. Medical and nursing education, he said, should be placed on an absolutely comparable basis. In the preclinical years the same instruction should be given to both groups. Only in the clinical period should specialization begin along different but equally substantial and supplementary lines. The future of the health of the nation rests upon the raising of nursing to this plateau, he argued, as well as upon vastly improved medical preparation.

The dean of a medical school asked incisively, "Do you suppose nurses *want* to carry trays? If they would only make up their minds about what they want to do!" A hospital director, whom the writer met early in the study, inquired if she had yet discovered that the "head nurse" is at once an administrator, a supervisor, and a teacher. "I can see," said he, "that she should have a college education." The head of a famous department of psychiatry wanted to know if the writer could give some indication of how soon he might hope to obtain nurses who would be "colleagues in research and writing."

When statements such as these are reported to nurse educators, many have a tendency to look almost incredulous. So accustomed are they to meeting clinicians and hospital administrators who are chiefly worried about the inadequate amount of general nursing care, that they scarcely realize that there are physicians, probably many of them, convinced that a new day must dawn for nursing education. Although there are numerous doctors who fail to see beyond the need for a large, readily available, and inexpensive supply of nursing service, there are other voices to be heard. Some of the most encouraging and truly forward looking help received by the writer has come from those medical educators, practicing physicians, directors of hospitals, and public health specialists scattered across the nation who view the future of nursing with faith and sympathetic interest. They are potentially the best friends that nursing education could possibly have. They should be sought out, their acquaintance cultivated, and their constructive assistance requested. The fact that many of them are men of great prestige who will be listened to by colleagues and laity alike, should be viewed as a distinct asset, not as a reason for timidity and hesitation in approaching them.

This introduction cannot appropriately be ended without some word of appreciation to those many persons, institutions, and organizations who have participated in this effort. Thanks should go first to the National Nursing Council, including particularly

Miss Sophie C. Nelson, chairman of the corporation, and Miss Marjorie B. Davis, its executive secretary. The Council not only planned and fostered the project; it has given the director whole-hearted moral support and encouragement. In addition, Miss Davis has carried responsibility for the administrative aspects of the study. Even when the days and frequently nights of work have been exhausting, her enthusiasm and graciousness have never flagged.

Thanks should perhaps go next to the foundations that have cooperated to an exceptional degree in making possible the preparation of this report. Appreciation is due especially Dr. Oliver C. Carmichael, president of the Carnegie Foundation for the Advancement of Teaching, both for his advisory assistance to the Carnegie Corporation in connection with its generous grant of funds, and for his continuing counsel. Appreciation is also due Miss Mary Elizabeth Tennant and the medical staff of the International Health Division of the Rockefeller Foundation for their many indications of interest and helpfulness. The writer wishes additionally to express appreciation to Russell Sage Foundation, which granted her leave of absence for the period of the study, bore part of its expense, and offered to publish the report.

To the Division of Nursing of the United States Public Health Service the writer is particularly indebted. It not only tabulated requested statistical data, prepared memoranda, and made available for examination much pertinent source material, but its chief, Miss Lucile Petry, and her staff gave entire days to exceedingly helpful and imaginative discussion of the future of nursing education. Similarly Miss Blanche Pfefferkorn, director of the Department of Studies of the National League of Nursing Education, and Miss Ella A. Taylor, statistician for the Department, permitted innumerable interruptions of their work in order to collect and check factual data without which the report would be sadly lacking.

23

To the members of the several committees, the workshop, and the regional conferences, the writer also expresses hearty appreciation for their help. For the hospitality extended her during her visits around the country, the writer is very grateful. She wishes particularly that the Catholic Sisters, who received her in their schools with a warmth and friendliness far exceeding the demands of professional courtesy, may know of her gratitude.

The writer's part in this study has afforded her an exceptionally rich opportunity to see and share in the on-going life of the profession of nursing, which is at once so old but in its professional aspect so new. She hopes that nursing education will soon be established on a sounder and more substantial base; that nurse educators will be able to look back on these years of struggle and uncertainty with wonder that the road could have seemed so hard, and able to look ahead with some gaiety of spirit, secure in the knowledge that theirs is a socially vital and a socially recognized profession.

E. L. B.

June, 1948

EXTENSION OF HEALTH SERVICES

ENLARGED and rebuilt hospitals, consolidation of hospitals, more hospitals! Those are the most obvious manifestations of the extension of health services. Architectural blueprints in large numbers have been completed; money is in hand or in sight in considerable amounts, thanks to the Hospital Survey and Construction Act of the Seventy-Ninth Congress and to action by hundreds of other public and private bodies and persons. Only the scarcity of building materials and labor, and excessive costs have delayed the construction program.

As a consequence of the distinguished work of the Commission on Hospital Care, which resulted in the publication of Hospital Care in the United States[1] and stimulated nearly all the states to create commissions for the study of needed hospital development, there are now available comprehensive data on the quantity and distribution of hospital facilities. The Commission concluded that an additional 195,000 general hospital beds and 45,000 beds for the care of tuberculous patients would be needed; that probably a quarter of all existing beds are in institutions where replacement or consolidation is requisite; that more adequate facilities for the mentally and chronically ill would presumably be indicated by further investigation. If any appreciable proportion of these beds is provided, the task will be no small one.

THE HOSPITAL AS A COMMUNITY HEALTH CENTER

But something more than mere building and rebuilding of physical structures is contemplated, both by the Commission on

[1] New York, Commonwealth Fund, 1947.

25

Hospital Care and by many persons in the Federal Security Agency and others who are concerning themselves with the hospital's social function. Supposedly this institution will become far more of a community health agency than at present. Within the general hospital provision will increasingly be made, it is believed, for the care of persons with communicable diseases; for convalescent patients; and for certain types of tuberculosis, and of nervous, mental, and chronic diseases; as well as for acute illness and injuries.

The importance of the outpatient department is being progressively emphasized. Transient illnesses, as the Commission notes, can be effectively treated there; diseases of serious nature can often be detected in incipient stages, and some of a chronic nature can be treated through therapy. Also "follow-up" service; immunization programs and well-baby clinics; mental hygiene, maternal, and other clinics; and teaching of health care are among the functions that can be carried on successfully by well-organized, administered, and staffed outpatient departments. As awareness grows of the importance of these functions and as new construction proceeds, hope appears that facilities more conducive to human dignity and to the teaching of positive health may replace the present cramped, dismal quarters often allotted to these departments, in basements or semibasements of hospitals.

Still further and drastic changes in transforming the general hospital into a community health agency are being recommended. The Commission summarized these proposed changes by suggesting that hospitals make their laboratory and other diagnostic facilities readily available to the members of the local medical profession, as well as to their medical staffs. Diagnostic clinics should be established in general hospitals in the interest both of the general practitioner and the patient. Office space should be made available within hospitals when conditions permit, and when such arrangements are desired by members of the

26

medical staffs. For the extension of group medical practice, hospitals are encouraged to combine their efforts with those of the local medical profession. Hospitals should arrange, wrote the Commission, for the use of their equipment and technical personnel "by organized groups of physicians" to the mutual advantage of patients, physicians, and hospitals.

This, then, is the over-all plan for the general hospital as it is being visualized. It will be far more inclusive in its intra-institutional functions than at present. But the general hospital is also being conceived of as related to other community health agencies to a degree previously unknown. It is portrayed as having its place and role within a *coordinated system* of health agencies. In a "pilot study" of the state of Michigan, the Commission probably did its most creative work. It fashioned a pattern applicable elsewhere on a statewide basis, or to localities where sectarian groups such as Roman Catholics, Latter-Day Saints, or Seventh-Day Adventists operate a number of geographically well-situated institutions.

The Commission viewed this new kind of general hospital as a regional hospital or medical teaching center around which would be grouped smaller community hospitals. These smaller hospitals, in turn, would have grouped around them local health centers designed to provide certain services to rural areas. In Michigan plans were drawn for two centers for medical education and service; 21 regional hospital centers; 81 community hospital centers; and 181 local health centers.

It was assumed that the two medical centers would have *large* hospitals and would conduct complete programs of medical, nursing, and hospital care. Their function would be not only to educate physicians and nurses and train technical personnel, but also to help maintain and improve the quality of hospital and medical care in the entire state through educational programs offered on a postgraduate and an extension basis. The Commission suggested that these medical schools send men regularly to

27

the regional and community hospitals, there to conduct clinics and seminars for the physicians practicing in the locality; that the schools make provision for skilled consultants to respond to calls for assistance from local hospitals.

The regional hospital centers, because of their size and location, would serve as focal points for the coordination and integration of hospital service over an area of several counties. In most instances their capacity was set at 200 or more beds, never fewer than 100. They were expected to provide special services that the smaller community hospitals could not afford to maintain.

Community hospital centers were viewed as those which, because of size or location, need hospitals of 50 or more beds. Public health and medical service centers were planned for places too small to justify the establishment of a hospital and yet sufficiently large or isolated to need an institution for medical service. These centers would supposedly function as branches of the county or district health departments, with offices for public health nurses. They might have diagnostic facilities for the use of local physicians who frequently would have their offices in the centers. They would be equipped to give emergency treatment, and might have beds for normal obstetrical cases. Ambulance service to the nearest general hospital could well be provided. The medical service would be under the administration of the medical staff of the hospital with which the health center was affiliated.

Through some such system of integration the duplication of facilities could be largely eliminated; plans could be made for the systematic inclusion and distribution of services not now furnished; and standards could be better maintained through provision for a flow of education, consultation, and services from the medical teaching centers and the regional hospital centers. It was believed, furthermore, that the establishment of community health centers would so improve the conditions of practice in rural areas that health personnel of all kinds could be obtained and held more easily.

Coordination was not to stop, in the opinion of the Commission, with the creation of working relations between general hospitals. Such hospitals would also be expected to coordinate their efforts with those of specialized hospitals and public health agencies. Scientific equipment and professional personnel in the general hospital could profitably be used to assist in the treatment of patients in tuberculosis sanatoriums, hospitals for nervous and mental diseases, and institutions for chronic and convalescent patients. Particularly heartening were the recommendations for bringing more nearly into alignment the philosophy and practice of the general hospital and public health programs. Said the Commission:

There should be close relationship between hospital and public health department programs so that the educational activities of the hospitals can include training in public health work.

Unnecessary duplication of effort and equipment should be avoided whenever possible through joint use of facilities by hospitals and public health departments.

Integrated action programs, involving laboratory tests, x-ray examinations, case-finding activities, maternal and child clinics, outpatient services, and communicable disease control, should be conducted jointly by hospitals and public health departments.

Cooperative programs of health education, preventive medicine, visiting nurse service, social service, and statistical reporting between hospitals and public health departments should be extended.[1]

Were it possible to devote further space to the question of the hospital of the future, the reports of prospective plans, made to the writer by various deans and professors of medicine and by hospital administrators scattered over the nation, would be recorded. These reports would constitute evidence of the intellectual ferment in many places. They would indicate that atten-

[1] Hospital Care in the United States, p. 30.

tion is beginning to be focused upon local areas needing cultivation, and local conditions needing improvement. They would demonstrate, furthermore, that the report of the Commission on Hospital Care, almost exclusively cited here in behalf of brevity, is not only a guide for, but a symbol of, planning that is confined to no one agency or to no one state. Obviously change will come at varying rates of speed and in different ways in different places. It appears obvious, however, that the massive walls which for so long separated the hospital from the outside world are beginning to crumble. The hospital is moving *out* into the larger community; the community is moving *into* the hospital. The implications are too large to be foreseen in their entirety.

EXPANSION OF PUBLIC HEALTH SERVICES

Other changes in the extension of health services are also foreseeable. Public health facilities are being rapidly extended, not only in the area of prevention but of therapy. States that have been in the vanguard of the public health movement have accomplished such impressive results in reducing morbidity, infant and maternal mortality, and mortality from communicable diseases that they are eager to extend these benefits. They want to attempt, moreover, to come to grips with those particularly destructive "diseases of middle life," such as cardiac diseases and cancer, and with the degenerative process of old age. Increasingly they see the significance of the role played by bad social and living conditions and by inadequate education in health matters. Hence they are in the process of strengthening their alliances with social welfare agencies and with the teaching profession. They view their teaching function as of paramount importance, and the school and industry, besides a wide variety of clinics, as fertile ground in which to carry it on.

More hesitant or economically poorer states have witnessed the accomplishments elsewhere, and have come to realize that they *must* attempt to catch up. As a consequence the postwar period finds the legislatures of many states receptive to granting funds for the creation or enlargement of official agencies. The dearth of well-prepared and experienced personnel, however, is badly retarding the progress of this dynamic movement.

If anyone questions the vitality of the interest in public health matters, he should note that although public health services are largely in the hands of state and local agencies, nearly every session of the Congress makes further provision for grants to the states. At present the federal grants amount to some $50,000,000 annually for work in the control of venereal disease, tuberculosis, and cancer, mental health, and maternal and child health.

Perhaps the greatest shortcomings of the public health movement are the proliferation of agencies; the overlapping and duplication of function on the one hand, and on the other, the serious gaps in service available. It is assumed that these difficulties must be realistically faced in the near future, and better coordination of effort achieved. The Commission on Hospital Care has indirectly pointed to its proposed solution of some of this trouble. Whether the public health movement will accept this solution of integration with the general hospital, or seek other means for reducing waste of personnel and funds and for achieving greater efficiency, remains to be seen.

LARGER FINANCING OF HEALTH SERVICES

The financing, as well as the delivery, of health services is a question of such magnitude that it has become a national political issue. Can ways and means be found whereby more health care can be made available both to families who have been receiving some care and to those who have received almost none? For nearly ten years Senator Robert F. Wagner has been seeking a solution through federal enactment of a compulsory health insurance bill. In recent years Senator James E. Murray and

Congressman John D. Dingell have shared responsibility with him. An alternative proposal, generally known as the Taft Health Bill, was introduced much more recently. It seeks to make federal grants available to the states for expansion of medical and dental services to low-income families and individual persons, without discrimination as to race, creed, or color. Relatively more assistance would be provided for economically poor than for wealthy states. Whatever may be the outcome of federal legislation drafted along these two divergent patterns, a comprehensive bill for the enlargement of health services is almost certain of ultimate enactment.

During the past decade while the Congress could not make up its collective mind about so large an extension of medical care, prepayment plans for hospitalization have met with notable success. Voluntary health insurance to cover partial medical and surgical care is being increasingly offered to the public. No fewer than 43,000,000 persons, it is estimated, are enrolled in some plan for hospitalization; 26,000,000 for medical and/or surgical care; 21,000,000 for weekly or monthly cash payments in case of disability.[1] It must be borne in mind that there is no such numerical coverage of different individuals as these figures might seem to indicate. A large, although unknown, number of persons are enrolled in two or more plans. Unfortunately most voluntary health insurance is now too expensive for families in the lower income brackets. It must also be remembered that many of the plans provide extremely scanty coverage of service, and emphasis almost everywhere is still limited to therapy and hospitalization in cases of acute illness.

In spite of such facts, the growth of voluntary insurance plans and the promotion by the American Medical Association, even though reluctantly, of prepayment for some medical and surgical services is clear evidence of the active effort being made to find a

[1] Research Council for Economic Security, The National Health and S. 545. Chicago, 1947, p. 6.

financial solution to the problem of the cost of medical care. As actuarial and organizational experience accumulates, it is assumed that the insurance principle, perhaps on both a voluntary and a compulsory basis, will be more efficiently and widely utilized and that coverage of services—made possible in part through the extension of group medical practice—will be greatly broadened. It is also assumed that attention to positive health, now sadly neglected, will be included.

MAINTENANCE OF HEALTH AS THE FUTURE GOAL

These developments, thus far noted, are indicative of the movement that is primarily concerned with organizational change and with the creation of an administrative and fiscal structure whereby the delivery of health services may be enlarged and facilitated. There are, however, other changes under way which are perhaps of even larger import for the future. They deal with the nature and the quality of health services to be rendered. Thus far, the major emphasis in medicine has been centered on organic disease. The teachings of preventive medicine, mental hygiene, and public health have progressively stressed not only the prevention of disease but the maintenance of health. Only slowly have the implications of these teachings made themselves felt on the medical profession at large; only in small part have they as yet competed with the physician's interest in pathology. But time has brought enough realignment of interest so that the dean of one medical school recently remarked that organic disease, as motivation for operating a medical school, had worn itself out and new motivation must be found.

The pendulum has begun to swing farther in the direction of health; of emphasis upon the "normal" person, and sickness as a deviation from the normal; of an understanding of the emotional factors which are a component—if not the cause—of disease; of the responsibility of the health professions in aiding persons,

33

individually and groupwise, to maintain positive health.[1] This responsibility, many are coming to believe, is the challenge and the new source of motivation for the years ahead.

Representatives of the laity, moreover, are beginning to aid the health professions in emphasizing this positive approach. The emphasis upon prevention of disease, wrote a clinical psychologist to the author, seems "to reflect a larger cultural trend in America, a growing recognition that we must conserve our resources, human and material, if our society is to continue. Perhaps it marks the end of an era of exploitation and rampant 'individualism,' and the beginning of a process of redefining the concepts of 'self interest' and freedom."

Where attention has been shifted toward these more recent principles, surprising results have occurred in the areas of medical education and practice, and similarly of nursing education and practice which will be viewed later. Because it is impossible to discuss all the changes that are becoming apparent, the following pages will be confined to illustrations taken from psychiatry, pediatrics, and obstetrics.

Particularly encouraging are current developments in *preventive* psychiatry. Until recent years the medical school made mental disease, like organic disease, the focus of attention. Lectures and clinical observations were centered on psychoses and psychotic patients. Psychiatry was a department usually quite separate from other departments of the school. Its function was limited to providing a little highly technical information of small

[1] Nursing in Modern Society by Mary Ella Chayer, professor of nursing education at Teachers College, Columbia University (New York, G. P. Putnam's Sons, 1947) contains three chapters that are particularly pertinent to the discussion of the maintenance of health. The Significance of Human Behavior, The Newer Approach to Child Development, and The Fundamental Concerns of Parents present an excellent portrayal of the manner in which a well-known nurse educator views this enlarged emphasis on health and the role of nursing in relation to it.

This book is recommended to the laity, for whom it was written quite as much as for nurses. The way in which nursing has been placed within the larger societal process clearly emerges from the titles to the three parts: The Impact of Social Forces upon Nursing; The Influence of Social Forces upon Community Health Needs; and Building a Better Future.

value to the general physician, and which more rightfully belonged to training for the specialty of psychiatry. Even before the outbreak of the recent war, the total inadequacy of such education began to be apparent. Conviction deepened as the medical profession struggled with the emotional problems of men in service or deemed unfit to enter service. As a consequence, reorientation or expansion of earlier plans is already under way in several institutions.

The function of psychiatry in the undergraduate medical school, agree the teachers responsible for change, is to provide *all* students with: first, a comprehensive understanding of the significance of emotional factors as a component or cause of sickness; second, relatively simple techniques for the treatment of emotional disturbances or neuroses in their early stages; third, diagnostic ability to recognize disturbances of a sufficiently severe or deep-seated nature to need referral to a psychiatrist. Where these goals are being sought, lectures on personality structure and human behavior are likely to appear in the first year of the medical school; much of the clinical instruction is not in the psychiatric service but in the medical outpatient and inpatient services; the psychiatric service is utilized more for comparative observation of pronounced deviation from "normal" behavior than for detailed study of types of psychoses.

As the medical school moves into its new orientation in this area, the question immediately arises of how similar information may be made available to physicians already in practice. Anyone who has read Dr. Carl Binger's forthright article, "Why the Professor Fell Out of Bed," in Harper's Magazine for October 1947, is convinced that if the war against neurosis is to be waged with any large degree of success every physician must be prepared to practice *preventive* psychiatry.

The practicing physician needs information; he needs opportunity for clinical experience under supervision. Perhaps most of all he needs "reconditioning" in his attitude and approach to patients. He must be taught to *listen*, for listening to his patient is, in itself, an important part of psychotherapy. But the time, patience, and concentration required by the listening process run counter to long-established habits of getting patients in and out of the physician's office or clinic with dispatch. One psychiatrist said half facetiously, "The hardest job I have is to teach the general practitioner that he is to sit in a chair for an hour, listen, and keep his mouth shut." In commenting on this remark another psychiatrist noted, "My colleague may succeed in persuading the practitioner to sit in the chair, but he will not succeed in getting him to keep his mouth shut."

Even in regard to the difficult question of what can be done for the busy practicing physician, initial undertakings are promising.[1] Experiments in brief but comprehensive postgraduate courses have met with excellent results. The physician probably was not fully reconditioned in a period of two or three weeks, but he gained appreciable knowledge of, and insight into, the emotional component of disease. Initial surprise and even inner disturbance ended in acceptance of the validity and power of those emotional factors he had so largely disregarded, and in acceptance of the fact that he must attempt to fill a more significant role. Further experiments of this and other kinds will, it is assumed, be tried. Such undertakings must pass the experimental stage as soon as possible, however, if desperately needed help is to be brought to the medical profession at large.

[1] This chapter was prepared before Teaching Psychotherapeutic Medicine; An Experimental Course for General Physicians, edited by Helen L. Witmer (New York, Commonwealth Fund, 1947), reached the writer's desk. Although reference is subsequently made to the book in the text, its importance must be stressed through the insertion of at least this brief footnote. The volume reproduces the formal teaching materials presented to the general practitioners by the several psychiatrists who conducted a two-week course. It also includes a considerable amount of the discussion that stemmed from these lectures and from clinical cases examined by the general physicians under the supervision of the psychiatrists. The book is almost indispensable to physicians, nurses, and social workers generally who wish insight into the emotional component of disease and into simple therapeutic methods. It is equally indispensable to those many members of the laity, interested in this most important subject, who have long wanted to know how the benefits of psychotherapy could be extended in the face of the paucity of psychiatrists. The very fact that the book contains few technical terms is an added asset.

Another development of equally large import, and closely related to that in psychiatry, is what the writer calls the "new pediatrics" and the "new obstetrics." Pediatricians made their appearance as specialists in the care of sick babies and children. Gradually emphasis has shifted until they are coming to be thought of as persons who keep children well. In some places their professional standing and prestige in the community already depend upon their success in preventing illness. With assumption of responsibility for the *health* of children has come a quickening of their perception of the influence upon the child of the emotional milieu in which he lives. Let there be tension, anxiety, friction in the home, and the emotional impact, they have learned, will be transmitted to the child. Let there be a lack of maternal affection, and trouble will be stored up for him.

Those who read Dr. Binger's article will recall the statement that among his acquaintances are a few pediatricians who almost never have a feeding problem in their practices because they know how to reassure mothers. "These men are able to allay maternal worries over thumb-sucking, masturbation, constipation, tantrums, and nightmares and, by so doing, help to stop these symptoms." One pediatrician on the staff of a large hospital, Dr. Binger notes, writes "T. L. C." on certain charts. The initials stand for tender, loving care, which he prescribes at regular intervals and in definite doses. "He is convinced that he has shortened illness and reduced mortality by this prescription."

As soon as pediatricians visualize their primary function as that of promoting health, they almost immediately sense the need for detailed knowledge of what constitutes normal child growth and development, as well as the role of environment and heredity in fostering or hindering that normal growth. So imperative is the want for this knowledge now becoming that some of the more advanced medical schools, which cannot command the use of the university's nursery school, are even starting to operate nursery schools for normal children within their teaching hospitals.

37

The staffs of some hospitals, moreover, are beginning to realize that they can and should attempt to offer the community service which extends beyond the scope of the private pediatrician, the well-baby clinic, and the care of sick infants and children. The writer visited a child development center on the Pacific Coast which is an integral part of a children's hospital that recognizes its obligation to foster the maintenance of health. This child development center offers an educational and therapeutic service available to parents of all economic groups and to children of preschool age. Its basic aim is to cultivate the healthy, happy growth of the child and thus to prevent the distortions which may lead to personal and social maladjustment in later life.

The staff of the center includes two full-time pediatricians, one of whom is the director, a clinical psychologist, a parent consultant, and two nursery school teachers. There is continuous interchange between the staffs of the hospital and the center on medical, psychological, and educational ideas relating to the growth and development of young children. This relationship is of the greatest value to both institutions.

The program of the center is threefold: preventive, remedial, and educational. The preventive work begins in the well-baby conference, a part-pay clinical service offered to the community by the hospital through this center. Here the pediatrician sees the mother and child at regular intervals. He not only checks the physical development of the infant, but has the opportunity to explain to the mother the nature of emotional growth and to help her create a wholesome parent-child relationship early in the baby's life.

The guidance nursery school is maintained for emotionally disturbed children whose parents recognize the need for professional assistance. In some cases it may be a specific habit of the child that requires correction; in other cases tension and anxiety as expressed in aggressive, hostile, withdrawn, or overdependent behavior need to be traced to their source. The nursery school program is flexible and adjusted to help each child work through his special difficulties. Children with severe, deep-seated behavior problems are not accepted, but are referred to a psychiatrist. Experience has shown, however, that ordinary difficulties respond amazingly well to the kind of group and individual therapy which the school provides.

Remedial and educational work with parents is regarded by the center as an essential complement to its work with children. Discussion groups are organized for mothers, and individual conferences with both mothers and fathers are arranged. These remedial and educational discussions, whether individual or group, help parents to recognize and to change such attitudes and practices toward their children as may have been factors in producing behavior difficulties. Much of the work accomplished is, however, preventive and in anticipation of problems which will arise in the course of normal growth. The response of the parents indicates that they are eager for understanding which will enable them to guide their children to a full and creative life. Both the demand and the need for this kind of treatment and education may perhaps be gauged by the fact that, for every child and his parents admitted, some ten or a dozen children must be refused because of the lack of space and financial resources and personnel.

The pediatric residents of the hospital share in conducting the well-baby conferences; under supervision they carry on the educational work with mothers and infants. This is a most valuable training opportunity, as it familiarizes them with the emotional aspects of child care and thus broadens their concept of the role of the pediatrician. The staff of the center also offers an educational program, through group discussions with resident pediatricians, student nurses, student occupational therapists, and student dietitians. Emphasis here is laid upon the importance of understanding the emotional as well as the physical needs of ill children.

The center has recently incorporated training for a limited number of physicians and public health nurses. These students observe the children at play in the guidance nursery school, are present at developmental examinations, parent classes, and staff conferences, and assist in the work of the well-baby conferences—thus acquainting themselves with all aspects of the center's program. Discussions with staff members help them to understand the meaning of what they are seeing, the reasons children behave as they do, the ways in which emotional development follows the sequence of physical growth, and the techniques used by teachers and consultants in helping to solve problems arising in parent-child relationships.

About the "new obstetrics" the laity has already heard something, particularly since the publication in 1944 by Harper and Brothers of Childbirth Without Fear, written by Dr. Grantly Dick Read of England. Although it is being practiced as yet in only a few places in the United States in any of the fullness of its inherent philosophy, its followers are convinced that the implications for the future are profound. Physicians interested in this area have a few basic principles that are the foundation of the techniques they have evolved. They consider pregnancy a normal process which, unless pathologic conditions develop, should be as normal and painless as any other physiological function. They attribute discomfort in pregnancy and pain in childbirth largely to fear that results from ignorance and "old wives' tales," and to lack of good physical as well as emotional tone. They believe it possible so to "condition" mothers and fathers for the event of childbirth that both pain may be greatly decreased, and the mother's recovery and her ability to nurse the baby may be greatly facilitated. Those with psychoanalytic orientation believe, furthermore, that parents can be prepared not only to care adequately for the physical needs of the baby but perhaps to accept parenthood without the anxieties and tensions that are found in many families.

Teaching and the creation of a relaxed, friendly, and interested atmosphere are the cardinal processes used for translating these principles into practice. Early in pregnancy the attempt is begun to establish an emotional relationship between the physician or visiting nurse and the prospective parents, whereby the latter will feel continuing confidence and reassurance. The mother receives the best physical care that the obstetrician can give; she may in addition have the assistance of a physical therapist. But equally important is the aid given her, and preferably the father too, through personal interviews, literature, and attendance at discussion groups for expectant parents. Over the period of nine months the parents are made interested in the process of embryonic development; they are informed step by step about what will occur next in pregnancy and during childbirth; they are taught the physical care of the baby, his emotional needs, and something of normal child growth and development. The teaching process continues even during uterine contractions and delivery. Then particularly the physician and nurse work most closely with the mother. They explain each detail of what is happening; they keep her interested and encourage her in the progress made.

Thanks to the philosophy underlying the new obstetrics and the new pediatrics, as well as to psychiatry which has greatly enriched both specialties, an opportunity has now been provided for a *continuum* in parental and child care that begins almost with conception and extends as far as adolescence. Obviously an alliance between persons working in these two fields is a logical next step. Already cooperative efforts are beginning to appear. But the implications of what has been achieved in these areas extend even beyond parent and child care. The lessons that have been learned in how to allay fear and hence reduce tension and pain; in how to make the teaching process an instrumentality for conditioning persons in *positive health*—these are lessons of paramount significance for all members of the health professions.

II

FUTURE DEMAND FOR NURSING CARE

THE preceding chapter has very briefly sketched the probable development of some of the health services of the future. Should current plans and trends grow to rich fruition, the result would be one of vast expansion of services, and also of coordination and cooperation of institutions and personnel in behalf of improved standards and greater efficiency. The result, furthermore, would be an interest to a degree hitherto unknown in the maintenance of health, rather than the repair of damage, as the goal of these services.

What are the implications of these potential changes for the nursing of the future? First and most obvious is the enormous supply of nursing care that will be needed if hospitals and public health agencies are to increase in number and size; if specialized hospitals for tuberculosis, and for mental and chronic diseases are to provide more active treatment; and if industry, municipalities, and other corporate bodies decide to broaden the scope of their health services.

Second and almost equally important is the greatly increased competence that will be essential to operate such health services. The fact has long been apparent that there are proportionately too few nurses prepared to give more than general bedside care. The efficient operation of hospitals, public health agencies, and other community health undertakings has been hindered because of the paucity of nurses with sufficiently broad educational and professional background to staff the clinical specialties; to plan, administer, and supervise large and intricate nursing services; to carry on the teaching functions necessary both for the public, including sick patients, and for nursing personnel. If expansion and development of health services, such as have been pictured above, are to occur, these current difficulties will have to be overcome at the earliest possible moment.

But what will happen in the event of another possible, severe economic depression, should there be still larger numbers of nurses, some of whom have had prolonged and expensive preparation? This is the question raised by many registered nurses (R.N.s) who are still threatened by the remembrance of the serious unemployment of nurses in the early 1930's. Even should there be a marked recession, demand for nursing care has been raised to so much higher a plane that a very large supply would probably still be needed. At that time relatively few general duty nurses were employed by hospitals. In fact, in 1932 only 37 per cent of all hospitals connected with schools of nursing had any nurses in that category. Private or special duty nurses and student nurses constituted the great majority of the nursing personnel. With the onslaught of the depression, the demand for private practitioners declined sharply. They had little preparation for entering other fields of nursing, even if such fields had been developed sufficiently to require any large numbers.[1] Their situation was acute. Since then diversification in nursing services has shown as marked a growth as has the demand for nursing care. Consequently, the precarious field of private duty has become proportionately less important, while salaried institu-

[1] Because the private duty nurse has the opportunity to give her concentrated attention to one patient and usually has ample time available for examination of professional literature, it might be assumed that she would be in the vanguard of the best practices in nursing. Experience has shown this generally not to be true. Like the general practitioner in medicine, she tends to lag behind. By contrast, hospital and public health staff nurses work within a supervised environment where they see new developments, and are required to bring their practice in line with such developments. Furthermore, the trend, as indicated in the recommendations of the Commission on Hospital Care, is toward expecting the hospital to provide sufficient nursing care so that individual patients will not have to employ private duty nurses. In the light of these facts, younger private practitioners who wish to develop professionally and to enhance their security should probably prepare themselves for salaried practice in a clinical specialty. Nursing students, moreover, should be advised carefully regarding the disadvantages of private practice.

tional, public health, and industrial nursing has come to be largely considered a social necessity.

Hence the basic question for the years ahead, we believe, is whether a quantitatively and qualitatively requisite amount of nursing care *can* be obtained. In a recent report by the Women's Bureau of the United States Department of Labor, two estimates of the number of nurses needed to serve a probable population of 153,000,000 by 1960 were presented. In round figures they were 500,000 and 550,000.[1] These estimates, the lower of which is not far from 200,000 higher than the number of available nurses in 1946, represent requirements only if current standards of nursing were maintained. Were broader objectives sought, such as provision for more nursing care for mental patients and others than is now available, twice as many nurses would be required.

The Women's Bureau maintained that the 1960 figures could not even be approached if preparation does not proceed at a higher rate than any reached during the war. To reach the larger of the two estimates graduates from 1951 to 1960 would need to average over 45,000. In 1947, thanks to the subsidies provided by the Cadet Nurse Corps, graduates reached the impressive figure of 40,700.[2] Thereafter, however, a sharp drop was to be expected. In the same year that saw this largest number of nurses ever graduated, admissions to the 1,253 state-accredited schools totaled only some 38,000, or an average of 30 students per school. Even these 38,000 admissions were achieved by the most strenuous recruiting efforts. Somewhat more than 30 per cent of those enrolled may be expected to drop out before completion of the three-year curriculum. Hence the number graduated in the class of 1950 will probably be fewer than 27,000. It must also be borne in mind that, if figures for annual attrition from 1930 to 1939 continue to be representative of the future, approximately

[1] Estimate of the Need for Professional Nurses, 1947–1960. April 1947, mimeographed.

[2] National League of Nursing Education, "Graduations and Withdrawals in Class of 1947," American Journal of Nursing, January 1948, p. 52.

6.33 per cent of the total number of active graduate nurses will leave the profession each year.

Recruiting continues on a broad scale. Specialists in public relations have advised about refinement of recruiting techniques. Nursing associations on the national, state, and local levels, and nearly all individual schools have actively campaigned for more students and have begged graduate nurses to remain in nursing. The American Hospital Association, the American Medical Association, and various state and local bodies of hospital administrators and physicians have tried to help. So have many representatives of the public. In spite of all attempts, there is little real hope that an adequate supply of graduate nurses can ever be obtained if demand remains insistent.

Present Conditions in the Practice of Nursing

Many thoughtful persons are beginning to wonder why young women in any large numbers would want to enter nursing *as practiced*, or schools of nursing *as operated*, today. The facts about nursing as the average R.N. is expected to practice it have been objectively and succinctly presented in "The Economic Status of the Nursing Profession," prepared by the federal Bureau of Labor Statistics from nearly 22,000 replies to a carefully devised and detailed questionnaire.[1] In October 1946 the average graduate nurse paying for her own living quarters earned between $170 and $175 a month. Not only the smallness of this amount but the lack of opportunity for promotion and salary increases was reason for complaint. The actual work week for nurses in all fields averaged forty-four hours. For institutional nurses scheduled hours rarely exceeded forty-eight, but about one-third of them actually worked fifty or more hours. Slightly more than

[1] The preliminary report by Lily M. David of this socio-economic study was published in issues of the American Journal of Nursing for July, September, and October 1947, and in the U. S. Department of Labor's Monthly Labor Review for July, September, and November 1947.

half of the nurses obliged to work extra hours received no compensation for this overtime either in money or free hours. Most nurses on evening and night duty received the same hourly wage as for day duty. About a quarter of the hospital nurse's time, furthermore, was found to be spent in bathing and feeding patients and in clerical and routine duties, many of which might have been performed as readily and efficiently by nonnurses.

If these facts appear rather grim, it must be remembered, that only about one nurse out of four, excluding those in private duty to whom no such plans apply, was protected by a retirement plan contributed to by the employer, and only industrial nurses were covered by provisions for unemployment compensation. Again not including private duty nurses, paid vacations generally of two but not infrequently of four weeks and one or two weeks of paid sick leave were customary. However, most nurses did not receive free hospitalization, medical care, or insurance. Under these circumstances it is little wonder that a widespread feeling of insecurity caused more nurses to express dissatisfaction with the lack of retirement and unemployment provisions than with any other aspect of their work.

But there are other difficulties besides those discussed in this report which militate against entrance into nursing, particularly institutional nursing. About them little has been heard as compared with questions of remuneration and physical working conditions. Yet these difficulties are very real, and their resolution or lack of resolution will undoubtedly do much to determine the extent to which women with more educational and social background and more independence of mind and judgment will decide to enter the institutional field.

Hospitals predominantly are operated on the authoritarian principle rather than that of a cooperative team relationship. The nursing service is caught between the authority exercised by the medical administration, on the one hand, and the hospital administration, on the other. Unfortunately the nursing service also tends to be highly authoritarian. Hence the individual nurse finds herself with little freedom of movement and of initiative for other than specified duties, even within that service of which she is a part. In an institution where planning is done at—and administrative orders are issued so largely from—the top, slight opportunity is provided the staff nurse to participate in policy formulation that, however simple, would give her the sense of being an active member of a team. Rarely, in fact, is she accorded so much as the prestige of being considered the colleague of the physician. She is primarily a person who takes and carries out orders. As a consequence she tends to develop those socially undesirable characteristics of subservience to persons above her in the hierarchical structure and of mastery over those below her.

Not long ago Miss Dorothy V. Wheeler, director of nursing service of the Veterans Administration, declared that she believed that job dissatisfaction, and not insufficient remuneration, was the cause of a shortage of nurses. "The nurses want to feel that they have a share in what the hospitals are accomplishing and are not just a small segment which takes orders. They want a part in matters of policy." Concerning this desire hospital administrators and physicians—as well as many nursing administrators—have shown little understanding. In the editorial which quoted Miss Wheeler, the writer, presumably a physician, replied:

If a nurse looks upon herself as primarily a professional person, practicing a highly respected profession, under the necessary and natural supervision of physicians, it is hard to understand what matters of policy she will be especially concerned with. If, on the other hand, as a consequence of the partial unionization of the profession, the nurse has now come to look upon herself as merely a member of a working group which, like other groups in the labor movement, must continuously assert and reassert their equality with management, or with capital, then this new concern with "policy" becomes understandable.

We cannot remember any time when nurses exerted any greater influence upon institutional policy than they do today.[1]

[1] "What's Really Back of the Nursing Shortage?" New York Medicine, September 20, 1946, p. 11.

This is the general situation in institutional nursing. It is not characteristic of public health nursing. Although salaries and provisions for economic security are not appreciably better in that specialty, the nurse occupies a position of considerable importance and responsibility in her own eyes and is accorded far larger respect by the medical and nursing professions and by the community. Neither is this situation characteristic of all individual hospitals. In numerous institutions salary and personnel policies are on so much higher a level that the administration—and perhaps the nurses themselves—would scarcely believe that the picture here portrayed is not grossly distorted. Those institutions clearly reflect in the quality of their nursing service the advances that have been made in realistic, progressive planning and more democratic administration of policy.

PRESENT CONDITIONS IN NURSING EDUCATION

Let us now turn for a moment to nursing education as it exists in the average hospital school the country over. Although this subject appropriately belongs to a subsequent chapter, some reference must be made to it here, because it is the school of nursing that plays a large part in determining who will enter nursing service and in what numbers. By no conceivable stretch of the imagination can the education provided in the vast majority of the some 1,250 schools be conceived of as professional education. In spite of improvements that have been made in most schools over the years, it remains apprenticeship training.[1]

[1] The Division of Nursing of the United States Public Health Service made an examination in 1944 of costs and income of 20 representative schools of nursing in various parts of the country. According to its figures, their costs totaled approximately $2,405,000. Of this amount, however, 66 per cent was spent on maintenance of students, and only 34 per cent on education. Income totaled $2,524,600. As an average for the 20 schools studied, 88 per cent of the income came from student services, 11 per cent from student fees, and 1 per cent from gifts and miscellaneous sources. Thus, although a few sustained a loss, collectively the 20 institutions which operated the schools made a small profit, and they simultaneously had student nurses available for much of the nursing care given patients.

48

Eighty-eight per cent of the students entering the basic program of schools of nursing during 1947 had not gone beyond high school. The enrollments of the schools ranged from fewer than 5 to 442, with a median of 73. Approximately 300 schools had fewer than 50 students. The reader may wish to conjecture about the quality of education that is, or can be provided, in such small teaching units, particularly when economy is a major consideration. The full-time faculty averaged three per school. Their preparation was totally inadequate according to any standards of higher education.[1]

In the typical school the first six months are devoted to classroom work in the physical, biological, medical, and social sciences, and in nursing and allied arts. What the high-school graduate acquires, other than intellectual indigestion, from so many subjects thrust at her in six months' time is something most educators would not like to contemplate.

Thereafter begins the clinical experience, if we may dignify with that term the supervised nursing service that the great majority of students are still expected to render the hospital. It has consistently been assumed that through *practice*—even if the supervision of that practice were often quantitatively and qualitatively inadequate, and prior classroom instruction were extremely deficient—the student would emerge at the end of three years a competent nurse. If practice made perfect, much could certainly be expected. In the typical school it runs to thirty-three hours a week during the remainder of the first year after the student finishes her preclinical training. During her second and third years, in more than two-thirds of the schools, practice

---

[1] Reports from 1,125 schools of nursing, participating in the spring of 1945 in the program of the United States Cadet Nurse Corps, indicate that 20,134 graduate nurses were engaged, predominantly on a part-time basis, in the administrative and instructional functions of these schools. Only 23 per cent had as much as a bachelor's degree in addition to their nursing diploma. Another 27 per cent reported that they were working for a bachelor's degree. A mere 4 per cent held a higher degree, and fewer than 2 per cent were working for such a degree. As might be expected, a large proportion of those holding a higher degree were found within the schools which received ratings from the Corps of "excellent" or "good."

(exclusive of time spent for planned clinical instruction, classroom work, study, and meals) is between forty-one and forty-
eight hours weekly.[1]

Regardless of its glaring inherent errors, the assumption about
practice does seem to presuppose that clinical facilities should at
least be adequate for the execution of that practice. Data, however, are available which demonstrate the extreme lack of clinical
facilities of the "home" hospitals used by many of the schools.
In 1946 the median home hospital had a daily average of 134
patients; one-fourth had 84 or fewer patients.[2] This figure could
profitably be compared with the several hundred daily patients
that a medical school considers requisite for the training of
medical students. When one views the figures for distribution of
these patients among the four clinical services considered absolutely basic for the preparation of nurses, the picture becomes
exceedingly unsatisfactory. In more than a thousand hospitals
reporting, 13 per cent had *no* pediatric patients and 76 per cent
indicated that pediatrics was their minimum service. Eleven per
cent had no medical patients or medicine was the minimum
service; 11 per cent were in the same situation regarding obstetrics, and 4 per cent regarding surgical cases.

When the daily patient average is below the minimum required by the state board of nurse examiners, schools in such
hospitals naturally must send students to other institutions for
affiliation, even in these basic services. Some schools, to be sure,
arrange for affiliation when it is unnecessary in order to maintain
state accreditation. For every school, however, that is more
generous than required by administrative rulings, several schools
undoubtedly attempt to provide training that is insufficient by
any except minimum standards.

[1] National League of Nursing Education, "Students' Hours of Practice per Week,"
American Journal of Nursing, March 1948, pp. 184-185.
[2] National League of Nursing Education, "More About Clinical Facilities,"
American Journal of Nursing, January 1948, pp. 50-51.

Lest anyone conclude that all hospital schools are like the average that emerges from these statistics, it must be said emphatically that the writer has visited some hospital schools that have traveled far toward being truly professional, both in their educational outlook and their accomplishment. These schools have achieved amazing results when their budgets, size of teaching personnel, and difficulties overcome are considered. They select their students and instructors with care; they attempt to integrate the preclinical and clinical teaching, and to enrich the entire curriculum with a philosophy of the social and health aspects of nursing; their clinical facilities are abundant and wisely utilized. There are other and more numerous hospital schools which, although less distinguished in their contribution, are nevertheless preparing nurses for general bedside care in a thoroughly creditable manner.

But such schools represent only a small proportion of the 1,250 state-accredited institutions. Many hundreds of hospitals still operate schools, as they have in the past, to avail themselves of the services of student nurses. Regardless of the improvements they have been forced to make by the trend of the times or their desire to attract students, their primary interest is not in education. Were such hospitals vitally interested in professional development, they would tomorrow relinquish their schools to auspices whose exclusive function is education.

Deterrents to Future Developments

We must conclude that the over-all picture of nursing practice and nursing education is one of drab monotony and blurred outline. The distinctive achievements of some forward-looking hospitals and hospital schools, public health nursing agencies, and university schools (to be discussed later) in bringing color and sharpness of line into the picture only tend to accentuate the otherwise confused drawing and unrelieved somberness of the palette. Is this a profession that would appear to attract women widely, to say nothing of men? Awareness of this situation has caused many physicians whom the writer has interviewed to ask almost rhetorically, "Would you have entered nursing?"

The progressive president of one medical college, within which are schools of nursing, dentistry, and pharmacy, long ago concluded that he would not be willing to have his daughter become a nurse as the school of his own institution was then constituted. He decided that changes should be made within the area of his responsibility. Whenever protests about these proposed changes arose from members of his hospital or medical staffs, he faced the members directly with the question of whether they would want their daughters to enter or practice nursing as it then existed. He believes that the question can now more nearly be answered in the affirmative in his institution.

Under existent conditions, the marvel to some is that so many women *do* enter, and continue to enter, this profession. The shortage of nursing care has strained patience and perspective to such a degree that there has been much recent talk of a very emotional kind about nurses not wanting to "nurse the sick," about their having lost all sense of service. We believe the facts belie such talk. Notwithstanding the acute shortage of nurses, there were nearly five times as many graduate and student nurses in 1940 as in 1910.[1] There are more in 1948 than there were in 1940.

It is true that more than 58,000 nurses were engaged in 1945 in administrative, supervisory, and teaching positions in hospitals and schools of nursing. But would anyone acquainted with the institutional structure of the hospital advocate decreasing still farther the administrative and supervisory nursing personnel, without whose services every hospital would be reduced to com-

---

[1] All figures here relating to supply and demand have been taken from Facts About Nursing, 1946, published by the Nursing Information Bureau of the American Nurses' Association.

plete chaos overnight? Would anyone want to wipe out the small instructional staffs that make possible, poor as a great many schools of nursing may be, the further training of nurses? It is true that about 21,000 women were employed in 1945 in public health nursing. Would society approve of weakening that much too fragile bulwark that has arduously been built against disease?

Who then is left to nurse the sick, as the public uses that term when it complains about the unwillingness of nurses to do it? In 1945 there were an estimated 59,000 full-time private duty nurses, 25,000 of whom were employed in hospitals. There were more than 69,000 full-time and 12,000 part-time general duty nurses. There were also more than 130,000 practical nurses, attendants, and orderlies at work in hospitals, and a large but undetermined number of practical nurses giving care in homes. Although far too small to meet the demand, these are nevertheless very appreciable numbers.

In traveling across the United States the writer has everywhere heard this question of willingness to nurse the sick discussed by nurses. About no other question perhaps has there been such consensus. Nurses both want and like to do bedside nursing, has been the almost universal statement. But they want an opportunity to give nursing care as they believe it should be given! The writer has talked to many nurses who had become tired and frustrated because they had been little more than hands and feet in constant motion, when they knew their patients needed someone with whom to talk, someone who could give sympathetic understanding. She will always remember, as a prototype of many others, the head nurse in a relatively favored hospital who complained to her bitterly each night that she spent in the nurses' residence, "Another day gone. I have run my feet off. What have I accomplished? There has been *no time to make patients comfortable*. I am completely discouraged and worn out. I simply can't keep on taking it, and so I'm going to marry the next man who comes along."

The writer concludes that the nurses are right: they do not dislike bedside nursing but only the conditions under which it is too often practiced. Hospital personnel is both insufficient in numbers and frequently lacking in efficiency or ability to work well within teams. In addition the organizational system of ward care that has evolved is so complicated, as will be seen in later pages of this report, that every day is filled with standardized procedures that must be carried out even at the expense of individualized patient comfort.

Unless women *do* like to nurse the sick, we can find no explanation for their continuing to enter this profession, with conditions of practice and education such as they are and with other occupations and professions very widely open to them. Time was when women had little choice except teaching and nursing. That day is forever at an end. For the young woman who wishes or can afford little preparation, there are clerical, industrial, and business jobs that provide more convenient working hours and as much remuneration. For women who invest in prolonged higher education, opportunity is almost limitless. "Do you know that women are now going into chemistry and mathematics, foreign trade, and public administration!" is the kind of remark that one hears with increasing frequency.

The basic appeal of nursing to women has until recently served the needs of the United States well; it is still serving them to a surprising degree. It is not now, however, capable of producing the large numbers of nurses demanded, and large reliance can scarcely be placed in it for the future, with opportunity elsewhere so greatly expanded, unless both nursing practice and nursing education are profoundly reconstituted.

Before turning to the problem of how nursing may be refashioned, a further word is necessary about the criticism that nurses have lost the ideal of service. Such an ill-advised remark would not seem to warrant an answer in this report. It happens, however, that the criticism points to something at the core of our national life which needs to be faced realistically if constructive planning even for the future of nursing is possible. There are many who believe, with what degree of justification we do not know, that much of American society has lost its former concept of service. Certainly there are too few persons with that burning passion for service that was displayed during the recent war by those conscientious objectors who worked as attendants in hospitals and who offered themselves for extremely unpleasant, if not actually dangerous, experimental research.

Whether in general the ideal of service be smaller or larger than formerly, American culture is certainly influenced to no slight degree by considerations of remuneration and prestige. Studies of other professions reveal that even the decision to enter a particular profession is determined in considerable measure by the possible financial gains and the status that may be expected. Once within the profession, its members tend to gravitate to places where opportunities for economic gain, pleasant living, and professional and social recognition are favorable.

As a consequence, there are still state hospitals for the mentally ill without a single resident psychiatrist. There are entire areas in which no pediatrician has ever opened an office. Society has bemoaned the absence of needed specialists, but it has rarely blamed them for not practicing in these places. It knows that changes will have to be wrought in the economic and living conditions of these spots before it can hope to have resident services. It has recently seen some such changes made within the federal hospitals operated by the Veterans Administration, and has noted the resultant rapid increase in the size and competence of the personnel.

Should more be expected in sacrifice of nurses than of doctors? Thus far the remuneration and status given nurses has been distressingly small. The federal government has been, as yet, the most generous employer. It pays the civilian nurses it employs the highest salaries; it accords officer rank to those in the armed

55

services. As for pleasant living, one institutional nurse in every five still lives within the hospital. Countless others occupy dingy, furnished rooms and eat in bad restaurants. If our common culture is to continue to place high value on material things, that fact must be solidly reckoned with in the building of a profession so basic to society as nursing.

III

DIFFERENTIATION OF NURSING SERVICE ACCORDING TO FUNCTION

WHAT then is a possible solution of this very difficult problem of obtaining a supply of nursing care that is quantitatively and qualitatively sufficient? Along with many other persons, we believe that the answer is inherent in the questions: What kinds of *nursing functions* need to be performed? Can persons be found and prepared to fulfill these *functions* effectively, whether they be graduate nurses or not?

One basic error, common to some other professions as well, has been primarily responsible, we believe, for the difficulties currently encountered. Emphasis has been centered upon "the nurse," or at best "nurses." The term as employed by the nursing profession and the laity responsible for making policy, moreover, has almost always meant the graduate nurse, the R.N., or the trained nurse as she used to be called. The fact that less economically and educationally advantaged persons often visualized a practical nurse when the term "nurse" was used has had little influence on the higher levels of thought and action. Had its influence been larger, at least the frame of reference might have been profitably broadened.

Emphasis, we are convinced, should have been placed squarely on *nursing*, and on *nursing functions* conceived of in their evolutionary and dynamic, not static, aspects. So long as attention is centered on the graduate nurse, no other avenue is open except that of the present frantic and probably futile effort to recruit more prospective R.N.s. Even appreciably better educational preparation is likely to be denied them, so insistent will the demand for nursing service continue to be. Once emphasis is shifted to *nursing*, however, several roads seem to point to potentially larger supplies of service and to possibly increased efficiency both on the nonprofessional and the professional levels.

Pressure of circumstances has been leading steadily toward those roads. Unfortunately the experience gained has not been sufficiently examined, assimilated, and fashioned into a philosophy for planned future action. For a long time two systems of nursing care have existed side by side. So fixedly, however, have eyes been focused on one of those systems—that of graduate nurses—that the other, if recognized at all, has merely received the designation of "auxiliary." Only recently and in a relatively small number of places have any profound efforts been made to fuse members of these two systems into *coordinated teams* in which each person, according to background, training, and experience, performs certain functions essential to total nursing care.

The System of Nongraduate Nursing Service

Practical nurses have probably existed for as long as persons have been hired to tend the sick. That they have often been highly incompetent because of lack of selection, training, and supervision, does not nullify the importance of the role that they have played in the home and that they can be trained to play far more effectively.

Because graduate nurses or larger funds are not available, attendants have provided the predominant part of the bedside care given in hospitals for the mentally ill, and for chronic, convalescent, and tuberculous patients. They even constitute the major part of the nursing provided the acutely ill in some large municipal and county general hospitals. Their technical skill and understanding of patients have ranged from extreme limitation to remarkable ability. However that may be, the important fact here is that they have been and are now the only considerable source for staffing groups of institutions that probably contain over one-half of all the hospital beds in the United States.

The orderly, moreover, has had a long career in the general as well as the specialized hospital, particularly in the care of men patients. That he, too, has often been inefficient and has performed duties for which he was unprepared without adequate supervision is no denial of the essential place he has filled. Within a well-coordinated team, with better in-service training, his efficiency could be greatly increased.

The practical nurse, the attendant, and the orderly represent the large core of the system of assistant nursing service. The past two decades, however, have seen the ranks of that system markedly increased and broadened. Ward maids began to appear in voluntary hospitals when student and graduate nurses were no longer willing to do so much maid service, and when the hospital discovered the economy in employing them for such work. Although they do not directly provide nursing care, they have freed large segments of the time of nurses to give that care. They are an indispensable unit of the personnel of every ward. Attendants gradually made their entrance into voluntary hospitals before the outbreak of the recent war. Routine duties such as the making of empty beds, the carrying of trays, and the doing of simple tasks for patients were assigned to them. They also provided an important instrumentality in releasing nurses to give medications, treatments, and other more truly nursing care.

Then came Pearl Harbor and the drastic stringency of subsequent years. In order to keep hospitals in operation a wide and often strangely assorted variety of personnel had to be employed. Receptionists, errand boys, ward secretaries, voluntary workers in and out of uniform, and helpers of many designations appeared in bewildering numbers. Assistant workers of the attendant type were sought far and wide; much less consideration than formerly was given to their national origin, marital status, or color of skin. Although the major field of the practical nurse had formerly been

59

private practice in the home care of the sick, every obtainable person so trained was pressed into hospital service,[1] or to a small degree into the hourly nursing service of a few visiting nurses' associations.

That many more hospital wards and health services did not have to be closed during the war for the lack of personnel is a tribute to the imagination and organizational skill demonstrated by administrators under exceedingly trying circumstances. It was tacitly assumed that once the war was over the hospitals could return to their "normal" ways, and that the voluntary hospital, at least, could get back largely to a graduate and student nurse basis. Like the producers of steel who have continuously insisted that in another six months the "emergency" demand would be over, many hospital administrators believed that presently graduate nurses would come trooping back and difficulties would end. The record since 1945 has demonstrated the error of that presumption. The bitter truth is slowly being borne in on those responsible for planning that, so great is the demand, there is no considerable body of nurses to come trooping back. Instead, they are being thinly dispersed over large geographic and occupational areas.

The task of the future therefore seems to be that of analyzing and utilizing the experience gained prior to and during the war for long-term constructive planning; of fashioning from those frequently inchoate elements a *functional* system in which, through coordination, training, and supervision, persons of many different skills may render efficient service in the area of the health services.

OBJECTIONS TO EXTENDED USE OF ASSISTANT PERSONNEL

In a 1947 pamphlet, Practical Nurses and Auxiliary Workers for the Care of the Sick, the Joint Committee on Auxiliary Nurs-

[1] A count for January 1948, made by the National League of Nursing Education of the number of hospitals operating schools of nursing which employ practical nurses, showed that about 25 per cent utilized this form of assistant nursing care.

ing Service, composed of appointed representatives of six national nursing associations, committed itself unequivocally to recognition of specific functions for assistant nursing personnel. In spite of this official statement, many individual nurses speak disparagingly of the use of assistant personnel in caring for the sick. In conversations with nurses throughout the country, the writer heard two recurrent arguments which indicate sincere anxiety: in one instance, anxiety concerning patient care; in the other, anxiety about the R.N.'s own future. Unless these fears can be allayed, the building of coordinated teams of health workers will be seriously retarded regardless of any official statements by joint committees.

Over and again directors of nursing service and nurse educators, generally employed in excellent voluntary hospitals, plead for the best in nursing service that can be provided patients. How can that best be available, they ask, other than through the exclusive use of graduate nurses? They often observe pertinently that even the giving of a bed-bath, the placing of a tray, or the drawing of a window shade may be made by the nurse into therapeutic elements in her care of an acutely sick person. They argue with absolute convincingness that the patient is, and hence should be cared for as, a complete or total person. Treatment of a localized disease or postoperative area is not enough. Treatment of the emotional component is equally important.

The reason that other persons plead for the use of a differentiated staff, particularly by the voluntary hospital that has usurped a large proportion of the supply of R.N.s, is that the best in nursing service that can possibly be provided is desired both for patients in *all* hospitals and in *homes*, and for the *public at large*. Were the personnel and funds available, such persons would like to see the finest individualized care supplied to every one, sick and well. The shortage of nurses makes it essential, in their opinion, that the existent supply be utilized more advantageously and distributed more equitably. The graduate staff

61

nurse should be freed, or should free herself, to the maximum degree from those relatively unimportant duties still performed by her in order that she may concentrate her whole attention, within the voluntary hospital, upon the acutely ill and those in greatest need of total care. Any private duty nurse who cares for one patient not in real need of her exclusive attention, and any hospital or physician who condones or encourages that practice, render a grave injustice to society.

Nursing care in most of the public specialized hospitals and many of the public general hospitals is on an extremely elementary and unsatisfactory level. At least enough thoroughly competent graduate nurses must be found for supervision, administration, and teaching both of in-service and clinical courses, and divisions of such hospitals used for clinical instruction must be adequately staffed below the supervisory level. Unless this can be done, little hope is seen for future improvement.

Furthermore, much thought is given to those 145,000,000 persons who are not recumbent in hospital beds on a given day. Very appreciable numbers of them need the home services of visiting nurses, which are not available even in much of urban America. Still larger numbers need active help in preventing disease and maintaining health.

Finally, those persons who advocate the use of a differentiated staff are not unmindful of that realistic problem of the individual's and the institution's budget. We are still far from discovering a financial method whereby the finest in nursing could be furnished to everyone in need. At least it is assumed that neither the patient nor the institution should pay for graduate nursing, if any part of that nursing could be done as efficiently by persons with shorter preparation.

Another reason for the lack of conviction by nurses about wide preparation and utilization of assistant personnel is apparently rooted in the fear felt by many private duty nurses of the trained practical nurse. They see in her a potential competitor who is much sought after and who often earns not much less than they earn. They do not like to think about the consequences, were the current demand for private practitioners to decrease or were large numbers of practical nurses "to flood the market." Even institutional nurses are sometimes alarmed about the latter contingency. They fear, so they say, that practical nurses may "take over." They refer not only to the capture of practice but to control of nursing policies.

That some practical nurses are even now in competition with individual private duty nurses can scarcely be gainsaid. Whether enough trained practical nurses could be produced to be numerically a source of worry to the profession appears exceedingly doubtful at present. That there would be any substantial future threat from them, should they become readily available, is still more unlikely *provided graduate nurses move in the years ahead to true professional status*. The test might eventually lie in whether real differentiation of function is achieved. The writer believes that a place of such responsible leadership can and should be given to the *professional* nurse that persons with trained skill in uncomplicated general nursing would be viewed by the professional nurse and by society as essential helpers, certainly not as competitors.

ENGINEERING AN EXAMPLE OF DIFFERENTIATED FUNCTIONS

The existence side by side, within an occupation one sector of which is professional, of several kinds of persons differing rather clearly in type of preparation and function performed, but not necessarily in name, has been so little noted by most persons that first encounters with the situation are often bewildering. Hence the experience of engineering may help to illuminate thought about nursing.

In its broad scope engineering is an occupation that employs persons with varying degrees of ability and training. It has within its ranks men whose training ranges from the most advanced scientific and technological education to very little formal education. Engineering enterprises require the services of three groups of men: professional engineers, whose primary functions are planning and directing; technicians, skilled in developing details of plans and in supervision; and engineering artisans, whose manual dexterity and experience are needed to carry out plans.

Professional engineers provide the intellectual leadership in engineering. Many of them are convinced, however, that there are not yet sufficient opportunities for truly advanced preparation so that the leadership is either as profound in scientific knowledge or in its understanding of social purpose as it should be. Because attention has been primarily centered on developing a general basic education within the undergraduate engineering college that would give the essentials of professional training to matriculants, graduate curricula have not been adequately cultivated.

Engineering technicians, who are generally spoken of as engineers and thus speak of themselves, are employed on the operating level. They do not confine themselves to engineering enterprises as do many professional engineers, but enter industrial production in considerable numbers. In industry they occupy supervisory positions in operating departments; they supply such technical services as drafting, designing, testing, and inspection; they fill commercial positions relating to the sale of technical products and services. Under no circumstances should it be assumed that these technicians are men of generally lesser competence than are professional engineers. Many of them have a specialized efficiency that amazes the professional engineer as well as the laity. Their work is of unquestioned importance in the maintenance and operation of industry and in the forwarding of engineering enterprises. The scope of their work, however, is narrow, and responsibility assumed for over-all planning and administration is negligible.

Trade schools and technical high schools are designed to provide training for engineering artisans. Many learn their vocation, however, by being employed on the job or by the in-service training furnished by industry. There are a handful of excellent technical institutes that prepare a relatively small number of technicians. Unfortunately these institutes are far too few to meet the large potential demand for technicians. The course of study is generally two years in length, and students are admitted primarily on evidence of their capacity, interest, and in some instances future employability, rather than on presentation of formal scholastic credentials. All curricula are more distinctly vocational than are those of four-year engineering colleges. Yet they include a substantial amount of the underlying and related sciences and usually some work in English and economics. "Doing to learn" is an important characteristic of the instruction; a considerable portion of the student's school hours is devoted to practice in laboratories, shops, drawing, and design. The ranks of this group are supplemented by men who work up from the artisan level, and by some graduates of engineering colleges who at least begin their practice as technicians.

The schools of engineering that confer degrees are especially designed for the formal training of professional engineers who wish to enter the fields of planning and management. The four-year instruction received in these schools is supplemented, during summer vacations and after completion of the academic course, by supervised practical experience in industry. Because of an imbalance in the proportionate numbers of engineering colleges and of technical institutes that arose from America's extreme devotion to academic degrees, relatively too many professional engineers and too few technicians have been prepared. Since the onset of World War II, professional engineers—like nurses—have been in urgent demand. Prior to that, however, many graduates of engineering colleges were obliged to take positions in the technical services for which their preparation had been unnecessarily long. At all times, on the other hand, the supply of technicians has been totally insufficient to serve the practical direction of industry.

BUILDING NONGRADUATE PERSONNEL INTO INTEGRATED SERVICE TEAMS

No one assumes that the task of creating efficient, differentiated but integrated nursing service based upon functional requisites will be easy or readily accomplished, or that progress will everywhere be uniform. No one who knows the diversity of conditions from hospital to hospital and from agency to agency would advocate a single pattern or even several patterns to be slavishly copied, regardless of suitability. What is advocated is wide experimentation, pooling and exchange of ideas, critical evaluation of accomplishment, and then further experimentation on the basis of lessons learned. What is advocated, furthermore, as an absolute antecedent to such experimentation is conviction, not lip-service alone, on the part of the nursing profession, the other health professions including hospital administrators, and the laity concerned with social change, that new patterns of nursing service must be evolved both in behalf of adequacy of supply and of quality. The elements for these patterns, it has been seen, are largely known. They have been used sometimes for years in differing degrees in many places. How various kinds of personnel can be better selected and trained, and their efforts coordinated is the problem to be solved.

Particularly instructive is an experiment now being undertaken in one large general hospital in solving the problem of unsatisfactory ward attendants. This hospital had been much impressed by the intelligence, understanding, and interest shown by the nurse's aides who had volunteered their services during the war. Could personnel be found and trained to replace the attendants, who would more nearly resemble these former volunteers? Public announcement was made of raised standards

66

for application and improved wages. In response to this request for persons designated as nursing aides, the hospital discovered among the large Negro community a hitherto untapped reservoir of personnel, well above the ward attendant group in intelligence and personality. Although the hospital is in a "border" city, it decided to select aides from among these applicants. One month of carefully designed and paid in-service training was provided as preparation for work in a particular division of the hospital. The aides were then assigned to that division. They were found shortly to be doing everything formerly done by ward attendants; they were also carrying, under supervision, an appreciable number of the more routine nursing duties previously performed by graduate nurses. So successful was the initial experiment that the plan, still less than a year old, has already been extended to several other divisions.

Space permits the inclusion of only one other illustration. Consequently, we turn to an experiment in total, integrated staffing of a teaching hospital that serves primarily as a diagnostic and surgical center for difficult referred cases. In this institution differentiation according to function has been carried far toward its logical conclusion. The women's wards, for example, utilize the services of ward maids, attendants, trained practical nurses, graduate nurses for specialized aspects of bedside care, sometimes student nurses, and ward secretaries. Each ward is administered by a head nurse who has had advanced preparation for, or considerable satisfactory experience in, ward management. She will presently be aided by two assistant head nurses, one of whom will supposedly devote her time to teaching both students and the regularly employed personnel. Particularly gratifying, in the opinion of the director of nursing service, is the transformation in morale and nursing practices on the men's wards. Gone is the orderly who had been far from satisfactory. Men attendants, men trained practical nurses, and men graduate nurses have been introduced.

Throughout the hospital emphasis is placed on the role each has to play as a team in the care of patients. Deviation from that role is believed to endanger good nursing care and team relationships, and also the carefully figured budget. It has been difficult, however, to persuade some graduate nurses that they must relinquish routine duties, the practice of which has become habitual. This plan of staffing was instituted during the difficult war period. At no time has it been possible to get or retain many of the persons desired. The results have been sufficiently good, however, so that the director is now having a careful analysis made of results obtained and next steps to be taken. It is to be hoped that a detailed description of this undertaking and a report of the analysis will be published at the earliest possible moment, in order that other hospitals requiring large amounts of specialized nursing service may be able to compare practices. Obviously so elaborate a plan is not suitable for the average community hospital where most cases are less difficult of diagnosis, treatment, and nursing care.

Before turning to a few brief suggestions about procedures necessary for attracting, retaining, and increasing the efficiency of assistant personnel in general, something more specific must be said concerning the trained practical nurse around whom so many hopes and also some fears center as the potential future source of much bedside nursing. Of the nongraduate personnel, she has had the broadest and most formal preparation, although it has rarely exceeded a year in length. Perhaps because she stands closest to the R.N., fairly specific policy determinations have been reached by the nursing profession about the area of her competence.

It was the consensus of the Joint Committee on Auxiliary Nursing Service and of the six boards of directors represented by that committee that the trained practical nurse "is prepared to care for subacute, convalescent and chronic patients and to assist the registered professional nurse in the care of others. She works under the direction of a licensed physician and the supervision of the registered professional nurse. She may work in homes, hospitals, institutions, public health agencies, doctors' offices, and in commercial and industrial firms."[1] The Professional Advisory Committee for the present study concurred in this statement and stressed the fact that the trained practical nurse might assist in the care of acute illness as the member of a team where adequate supervision was present. Such a statement of official policy, if widely distributed and staunchly supported, should do much to give recognition to the broad scope of the work available to her, and to her place within an integrated team at least in instances of acute sickness.

Unfortunately the trained practical nurse does not yet have any appreciable legal recognition and protection, which are requisite if she is to feel much assurance or pride in her job. Before she is employed by an institution or public health agency, her training will probably be carefully questioned. In the field of home nursing that is desperately in need of many thousand more trained practical nurses, however, she must compete—except in three jurisdictions—with any person who chooses to "nurse for hire." In some 20 states legislation forbids the use of the title, licensed practical or attendant nurse, to those who have not been granted statutory permission. But anyone may put on a uniform and simply call herself a "nurse." Only in New York, Arkansas,[2] and Hawaii have statutes been enacted which make it illegal for a person not a registered nurse or a licensed practical or attendant nurse to engage in nursing for pay. Under such circumstances one can imagine the chaotic conditions that prevail. The trained practical nurse who specializes in home care is likely to find that many of her colleagues in uniform are persons with no preparation and often little competence, but who succeed re-

[1] Practical Nurses and Auxiliary Workers for the Care of the Sick. New York, 1947, p. 7.

[2] Arkansas has provided no penalty, however, for violation by practical nurses of its nurse practice act of 1947.

markably well in passing as "nurses" and in collecting very substantial fees.

If such lack of regulation is detrimental to the building of a large body of respected and self-respecting trained practical nurses, it is positively dangerous to society. Numerous instances are known of techniques employed and drugs administered by well-meaning but ignorant "nurses" that endangered life. For the very reason that persons of limited education are most likely to be at the mercy of such a practitioner, it is doubly important that they be provided with any possible protection which they are unable to provide for themselves. Whenever efforts are made to end this disgraceful negligence through legislative enactment, loud cries proclaim that even poor nursing is better than no nursing. There are not nearly enough veterinaries to meet current demands; yet society requires that they be licensed before they can practice. Other means than mere avoidance of needed legal action must be sought for furnishing a more adequate supply of home nursing care. *We recommend that sound legislation relating to trained practical nurses be enacted promptly in states without statutes; that such legislation elsewhere be reviewed, amended, and made mandatory as of a fixed date.*[1]

Because this report concerns itself primarily with a very different topic, further discussion here of the practical nurse is impossible.[2] Attention must therefore be directed again to the total group of nongraduate personnel who perform or could be trained to perform the less complicated nursing duties. Surely the writer can offer no specific formulas for their recruitment and retention

[1] Unfortunately space does not permit discussion in this report of legislation and administrative regulations concerning nursing practice by, and nursing education for, other types of nurses. Hence it can only be stated emphatically that statutory and administrative review, amendment, and enactment of new legislation and rulings are reported to be needed in practically every jurisdiction. Many clauses in existing acts and many interpretative rulings of state boards of nurse examiners have become so outmoded that they are a serious obstacle to much needed developments.

[2] Now available elsewhere, however, is the first detailed study of this very important subject: The Practical Nurse written by Dorothy Deming, R.N., consultant in public health nursing to the American Public Health Association, and published in 1947 by the Commonwealth Fund in New York.

or for making them efficient in their work. Past experience nevertheless has indicated certain broad steps that must be taken if these *desiderata* are to be achieved. More careful planning and administration of policies as agreed upon should be instituted. Policies for selection, tenure, wages, duties to be performed, physical conditions of work extending to just such small but important details as adequate rest rooms, and so on, need thoughtful definition. Once determined these policies should be made generally known. If generously conceived to raise the importance and dignity of the nongraduate position, they would probably be of very appreciable help in recruiting personnel.

In-service training would unquestionably have to be fashioned into a truly effective instrumentality for initial and continuing preparation of personnel. Although it has long been used in hospitals, particularly in those which have depended largely upon attendant care of patients, there is wide consensus that its great potentialities have rarely been envisioned. Even industry, which has relied upon this form of training to no inconsiderable degree, is convinced that cultivation still falls far short of inherent possibilities.

We believe that in-service training should be at least as carefully devised and the quality of instruction as adequate as is training now given to student nurses in the typical hospital school. We believe, furthermore, that in-service training, rather than the operation of a school for the preparation of graduate nurses, should progressively come to be the essential task of the majority of hospitals. As will be argued later, other institutions can better prepare the graduate nurse than can they. At present many hospitals are sacrificing the area that they probably should cultivate assiduously to programs for student nurses which they are ill-equipped to provide.

In-service training, moreover, is needed by nearly everyone employed, graduate as well as nongraduate, on a continuing basis. Thus far its principal use has been to induct new, nongraduate personnel into their initial duties. It can provide considerable initial efficiency to be sure, but it can also be used to maintain and raise that efficiency. (Through it other evidence besides length of "satisfactory" experience is available for upgrading in salary and status, with the probable concomitant effect of producing a better satisfied as well as more efficient staff.) That in-service training, by whatever name called, is almost equally essential for graduate nurses can scarcely be denied. In a field where new scientific knowledge, new technical procedures, and new attitudes concerning the larger functions of the health services appear in rapid succession, failure to make provision for systematic examination of these developments is likely to handicap not merely the nurse but the institution or agency utilizing her services.

Perhaps most essential of all, if assistant personnel are to be recruited and retained, is the effecting of change in the emotional climate within which these persons work. So bad is that climate now in many places that the writer recalls the comment of an administrator in a representative community hospital. "We get practical nurses, they stay a few days or weeks and leave. You can scarcely blame them. They have no status. They are treated like scrub women." Unless attention can be centered squarely upon the importance of the contribution that each person brings to the health services, be that person ward maid or director of nursing service, efforts to create and stabilize a differentiated personnel will be of small avail. And unless every contributing person can be conceived of and treated as the member of a unified team, whose sole collective function is the cure of sickness and the preservation of health, we shall be little better off than at present.

We believe, therefore, that consideration should be given not only to provisions for greatly expanded and improved in-service training and for more carefully designed policies for recruitment and employment, but that primary consideration should be placed upon achieving better interpersonal relationships within the hospital.

72

IV

THE FUTURE ROLE OF THE PROFESSIONAL NURSE

IF NONGRADUATE personnel come to be utilized more extensively and effectively, the implications for graduate nursing will be profound. On the one hand, nurses will be given a better opportunity to devote themselves to those aspects of clinical practice that require true professional skill; on the other, still more will be expected of them than now in supervisory, administrative, teaching, writing, and research roles. At this point we wish to quote, with only very slight editorial change, a few paragraphs prepared by the workshop,[1] to which reference was made in the Introduction. The writer believes that nurses will agree that this definition of "the professional nurse of the future" provides a vista of the place of the graduate nurse both within nursing and within our larger society.

It is the opinion of this group that in the latter half of the twentieth century, the professional nurse will be one who recognizes and understands the fundamental [health] needs of a person, sick or well, and who knows how these needs can best be met. She will possess a body of scientific nursing knowledge which is based upon and keeps pace with general scientific advancement, and she will be able to apply this knowledge in meeting the nursing needs of a person and a community. She must possess that kind of discriminative judgment which will enable her to recognize those activities which fall within the area of professional nursing and those activities which have been identified with the fields of other professional or nonprofessional groups.

She must be able to exert leadership in at least four different ways: (1) in making her unique contribution to the preventive and remedial

[1] See p. 16.

aspects of illness; (2) in improving those nursing skills already in existence and developing new nursing skills; (3) in teaching and supervising other nurses and auxiliary workers; and (4) in cooperating with other professions in planning for positive health on community, state, national, and international levels.

To understand the characteristics and aptitudes which are needed by the effective professional nurse, it is necessary to visualize her in action against the backdrop of a rapidly changing and increasingly complicated civilization. In past eras nurses, like other groups, have often been expected to fit into traditional niches in a relatively static situation. In that kind of society the nurse might fill her place satisfactorily if she were a passive, obedient, and unquestioning individual. In a rapidly changing world the nurse's activities will require that she be alert and self-directing. The professional nurse must be able to evaluate behavior and situations readily, and to function intelligently and quickly in response to their variations. She must recognize physical symptoms of illness which are commonly identified with organic changes. She must also recognize those heretofore less considered manifestations of illness such as anxieties, conflicts, and frustrations, which have a direct influence on organic changes and are now thought to be the result of an incompatible interaction between a person and his environment.

Nurses in their longer contacts with individuals have more opportunities to observe behavior and to listen to expressions of thought under varying conditions than do physicians whose contacts are necessarily intermittent and brief. For this reason the nurse must be able to direct her actions and her verbal expressions on the basis of a sound understanding of human behavior and human relationships. If the nurse does not have this quality of understanding and cannot use it to deal effectively with persons, she may contribute to illness or counteract the efforts of other professional workers.

This then is the task, as the workshop visualizes it, that lies ahead of the professional nurse. Let us turn momentarily to the definition of nursing set down by Sister M. Olivia of Catholic University of America.[1]

Nursing in its broadest sense may be defined as an art and a science which involves the whole patient—body, mind, and spirit; promotes his

[1] Aims of Nursing Administration. Washington, School of Nursing Education, Catholic University of America, 1947, p. iii.

74

spiritual, mental, and physical health by teaching and by example; stresses health education and health preservation, as well as ministration to the sick; involves the care of the patient's environment—social and spiritual as well as physical; and gives health service to the family and community as well as to the individual.

Both the description of the function of the professional nurse formulated by the workshop and that of nursing formulated by a leading Catholic nurse educator are alike in their portrayal of nursing as something so broad in scope and profound in nature that technical competence is only one of its components. Technical competence alone would not supply that discriminative judgment, that alert self-direction, that skill in directing word and action on the basis of an understanding of human behavior and human relationships, to which the workshop points. Certainly technical competence would never enable the nurse to minister to the spiritual health and the spiritual environment which Sister Olivia emphasizes. Yet it is these very plus values, under whatever names given them, that leaders of the nursing profession since the days of Florence Nightingale have held truly essential. It is these values that raise nursing from the level of a craft to that of a profession; that distinguish the professional nurse from the person whose almost exclusive preoccupation is with the prescribed physical care of a sick person.

That large numbers of graduate nurses are not professional nurses within this larger meaning is obvious. How could they be when one recalls the narrowness and the poverty of the training provided them? Frequently their competence is no greater than that which should be possessed by the well-prepared practical nurse, because opportunity for growth and development in those broader aspects of professionalism has been denied them.

In spite of this fact the term "professional nurse" is now used by nurses almost interchangeably with graduate or registered nurse, and all schools above the level of those that prepare practical nurses are popularly called professional schools. As the workshop notes, this practice "has created confusion in the minds of the public and nurses alike concerning expected qualifications."[1] The writer wishes to add emphatically that, in her estimation, *this confusion results in grave injustice to society, to the nursing profession, and to those individual nurses who have struggled to become and are truly professional.*

A generation ago Dr. Abraham Flexner set down certain criteria for judging whether an occupation has attained professional status or not. According to his interpretation of the professions: (1) they involve essentially intellectual operations accompanied by large individual responsibility; (2) they are learned in nature, and their members are constantly resorting to the laboratory and seminar for a fresh supply of facts; (3) they are not merely academic and theoretical, however, but are definitely practical in their aims; (4) they possess a technique capable of communication through a highly specialized educational discipline; (5) they are self-organized, with activities, duties, and responsibilities which completely engage their participants and develop group consciousness; and finally (6) they are likely to be more responsive to public interest than are unorganized and isolated individuals, and they tend to become increasingly concerned with the achievement of social ends.[2]

Nursing has moved far enough in the direction of meeting these criteria so that it may be considered a profession, or at least an evolving profession. But for it to designate the 1,250 schools and all nurses who have been admitted to practice by the several states as professional, when only a fraction of the schools and their graduates can as yet meet the tests of professionalism, greatly lowers the prestige of nursing. The custom, moreover, provides

---

[1] So disturbed is the administrative head of one national nursing association about the indiscriminate use of the term "professional nurse," that she always refers to the nurse who is professional in the generic sense of the word as "the professional woman in nursing."

[2] "Is Social Work a Profession?" Proceedings of the National Conference of Charities and Correction, 1915, pp. 576–581.

the public with no greater assurance of competence than the often meager qualifications demanded by state boards or nurse examiners. Finally, this habit probably deters many young women of larger educational background from entering a field where so little distinction exists between persons with the most circumscribed preparation and those with truly professional education.

Hence we recommend that the term "professional," when applied to nursing education, be restricted to schools (whether operated by universities or colleges, hospitals affiliated with institutions of higher learning, medical colleges, or independently) that are able to furnish professional education as that term has come to be understood by educators.[1] Such schools as can meet certain defined standards should be designated as "accredited professional schools" and a list of them should be published at frequent intervals for distribution to nurses, the public, and particularly to prospective students of nursing.

We recommend, further, that the term "professional," when applied to nurses, be restricted to those who have been graduated from schools designated as professional, or whose right to be thus considered has been demonstrated through some system of examination; achievement that has been objectively evaluated, such as marked excellence in clinical practice, supervision, administration, teaching, or scientific research and writing; admission to fellowship in an academy of nurses; or by means of other plans devised to raise the status of nursing.

Lest graduate nurses who could not qualify as professional fear that this reorientation would work great hardship on them, it should be said that the number of professional nurses in the immediate future would not be large enough, in the face of demand for nursing service, to provide any effective threat to employment.

This step, already long overdue, is requisite if the profession is to move from adolescence toward adulthood. By taking the step

[1] Careful consideration should be given to the fact that professional schools in most other fields have already come within degree-conferring institutions to such an extent that possession of a degree is fast becoming a criterion of a person's having received professional as contrasted with vocational training.

notice would be served to a now dissatisfied public that nursing was really attempting to set its house in order; that it was seeking to profit from the experience of older professional groups; that it was striving to create a plan that would attract women with the ability, education, and interest necessary to serve the more complex needs of people, whether sick or well.

THE CLINICAL NURSE AS SKILLED TECHNICIAN

The functions of the professional nurse both in clinical practice and in the nursing specialties must now be examined in more detail. Attention will be particularly centered upon several continuing difficulties that need to be removed if this type of nurse is to achieve the social effectiveness the workshop deemed essential.

In clinical practice two distinct but interrelated kinds of functions have been most widely accepted as appropriate for the professional nurse to perform. One is the role of physician's assistant in carrying out technical procedures and treatments generally considered too complex or too dangerous to be entrusted to assistant personnel or to graduate nurses with only limited clinical training. The other is responsibility for critical observation of the patient, care of him sometimes for long periods without specific directions from the physician, and decision as to what should be reported, and when, to the doctor concerning the patient's condition. For the fulfilling of these functions larger responsibility is constantly being reposed in the nurse, although often neither the medical nor nursing profession is completely aware of the fact.

A few years ago Dr. W. T. Sanger, president of the Medical College of Virginia, became so interested in the implications of his observation that physicians were expecting graduate and even student nurses to perform procedures formerly carried out only by doctors that he asked the dean of the School of Nursing of his

78

institution to prepare a list of some of these procedures. Dean Sybil MacLean's unpublished report noted 17 procedures, such as the taking of blood pressure and the giving of intradermal, intramuscular, and (in some institutions) intravenous injections. She listed no fewer than 24 other procedures in which the nurse aids the physician, and is responsible for the arrangement of equipment and for the care of the patient following treatment. Finally, she noted those many techniques that the nurse was expected to teach the patient, like insulin administration, urinalysis for sugar and albumin, care of the new-born, and formula preparation.

These are tasks that are now considered to be squarely within the province of the graduate and student nurse in many hospitals. Almost certainly the physician will not wish to take them back. Almost equally certain is it that he will attempt to hand over to nurses further procedures as they are perfected.

The public understandably knows little of the skill, time, and judgment required to perform these procedures. To give the reader some sense of the nurse's preoccupation with them, in addition to those other necessary duties that must be performed, a few paragraphs will be cited from the report by Clare Dennison of a spot study that was made three times for twenty-four hour periods at two-month intervals in a large teaching hospital. Although many of the technical terms may be unfamiliar to the lay reader, he will not fail to grasp the number, variety, and frequent complexity of the procedures and treatments. More importantly, he will get some feeling, as he could not from examining the list prepared for Dr. Sanger, of the exigency of situations within which nurses must often work and of the instant responsibility that must be assumed.

In this study the operating, labor, and delivery rooms, and the outpatient and emergency departments were excluded. So were all diagnostic and research tests. Nevertheless, about one hundred different procedures and treatments were found, covering periods of time that ranged from approximately two minutes "as in taking the apex pulse to twenty-four hours of constant attendance as in watching patients in respirators."

From an average of 473 patients, 109 were ordered blood pressures in intervals of every fifteen minutes to once a day. Sixty patients, or one patient in every eight, received parenteral fluids or transfusions, and while these were not done by nurses, they required the help of a nurse and on two of these days patients were receiving continuous intravenous fluid and required constant attendance. The nurses gave gavages, placed fifth leads for electrocardiograms, and applied suction to surgical wounds, tracheotomies, chest cavities and throats.

They managed the apparatus for Wangensteen suction, tidal irrigation, and bladder decompression. They irrigated eyes, cecostomies, colostomies, draining wounds, urethral and ureteral catheters. They gave colonic irrigations. They did artificial respiration in the interval needed to obtain a respirator, and then started the operation of the respirator. They applied sterile compresses and painted lesions. They did approximately 230 dressings in a day, and this does not include the times these dressings were taken down to show the wound to a surgeon. They did catheterizations, sitz baths, and turpentine stupes. They used the Danzer apparatus. They gave insulin and taught the patient or his relatives to give the drug and examine urine. They administered approximately 1,500 medications daily, by mouth or hypodermic. They had an average of seven patients a day under oxygen therapy and specialed patients after craniotomies, tracheotomies, and the usual surgery. They assisted with lumbar punctures, thoracenteses, paracenteses, and phlebotomies.

While all this went on, they met the usual expectations of the staffs. They knew, night or day, without direction, what to watch for and report for the thyroidectomies, the breast amputations, and the prostatectomies. In general, it was not necessary for the surgeon to give specific directions nor to see his patient for several hours after the operation. It was not necessary to tell the head nurse to watch for any toxic symptoms, even after chemotherapy; it was taken for granted that all this would be done. It was understood that the nurses would know how to administer any drug—and pick up any error in writing the order. They would not be exonerated from responsibility if by error 4 cubic centimeters of belladonna were written instead of .4 cubic centimeter, and any nurse followed the written order. The nurses would have been condemned if a patient scheduled for a cataract operation went to the operating room with even slight symptoms of a cold—or if any patient went there with a premonition that he was going to die. It was not a simple matter to decide on the evidence of symptoms shown whether or not to call the doctor at 2:00 A.M., or to calculate to a nicety the time the doctor should be called in order to appear in the delivery room at the proper moment, but the right decision was usually made. It would have been very inconvenient for all concerned during those days if the nurses had not known a good deal about the apparatus used in orthopedics, the machinery of the respirators, the oxygen tents, and the suction machines, but the fact that they did know was probably never noticed, so long have nurses been considered an extension of all the services in the hospital. In addition to this, each nurse accepted the responsibility for all services rendered her patient by any subsidiary worker, and every minute of every twenty-four hours the nurses were responsible for the prompt observation and reporting of any change in the condition of any patient.[1]

Certain important considerations emerge from Miss Dennison's facts. Most obvious is the wealth of clinical material and of sound classroom and clinical instruction necessary if students are to learn to carry out many of these procedures, and to have the scientific knowledge and judgment that are absolute prerequisites to complex clinical nursing. Schools in hospitals with inadequate facilities and instruction are totally unable to prepare nurses for practice as it is now done in the larger institutions. Such schools can only prepare for the very limited nursing service required by their own hospitals. As a consequence thousands of nurses find themselves at a distinct disadvantage if they attempt to move into more complicated situations.

A particular hospital was being visited where a supposedly experienced nurse had just been added to the staff. It was discovered that she did not know how to take blood pressure, a procedure that began to be handed over to nurses during World War I and has been more widely placed in their hands than almost any other. In-service training can perform an essen-

[1] Dennison, Clare, Maintaining the Quality of Nursing Service in the Emergency. Reprinted from the American Journal of Nursing, July 1942, pp. 3–4.

tial function in remedying some such deficiencies, and particularly in teaching new procedures and treatments as they develop. But let no one think that nursing as practiced today through highly scientific techniques—and as it is likely to be more widely practiced tomorrow—can be done with justice to patient or to nurse on the basis of the training still provided in some hundreds of existent schools of nursing.

But there is another consideration of larger proportions, to which brief reference was made earlier in the report, that appears from this statement. The reader is likely to conclude that the nurse's day must be almost totally occupied with technical procedures, treatments, and recording. When does she have "time to make patients comfortable" in more than the physical sense? Although the above picture is somewhat distorted for the reason that technical aspects of nursing were under chief consideration, it is true that the institutional staff nurse in probably the large majority of places is primarily engaged in physical care. Unfortunately the philosophy of essentials of patient care that has evolved from public health nursing, mental hygiene, social casework, the newer psychiatry, pediatrics, and obstetrics, or psychosomatic medicine has yet exerted but restricted influence over general duty nursing.

Visit those hospitals where a graduate or student nurse is detailed to give medicine to each patient for whom it has been prescribed the length of the ward, and where other nurses are detailed to give treatments. Who is detailed to sit beside patients, except possibly on the pediatric service, and give a form of nursing care that may be more important than medicine or treatment? Visit those institutions where ward nursing is done not by functional assignment but by the supposedly more individualized case assignment. Even there the nurse generally has so many patients for whom she is responsible that such supportive care as is extended to them must be provided while she is figuratively "on the run." Yet the thoughtful director of nursing service in a vast teaching hospital was concerned about the need for more expert physical care to such an extent that she recently included in her unpublished annual report the following paragraphs:

Quality of nursing care cannot be measured simply by whether or not separate therapeutic measures have been carried out specifically as ordered. A basic requirement for good nursing is that it must be individualized, that it must include sensitivity to, ability to respond to and deal with the mental and emotional reactions which accompany physical aspects of illness; that it must help the patient to understand his illness, plan to regain his health, or adjust to his limitations. No matter how full may be the provision for covering these latter points in the physician's conferences with the patient, it is the nurse who is with the patient at all hours of the day and night and must meet situations and answer questions which cannot be escaped. These things are essentials of nursing care.

Trends in the care of specific medical conditions give new emphasis to the importance of individualized nursing care; for instance, newer concepts of maternal and infant care, getting away from rigid feeding schedules, the importance of a relaxed obstetrical patient before delivery, an increase in the recognition of psychosomatic conditions, the importance of mental hygiene in all care. These trends in medical care must be paralleled in nursing care.

A letter from an obstetrician with psychoanalytic orientation points to the nurse as "the tender and gentle link that exists between the patient, her illness and her healing process." In his opinion "too many nurses and physicians are amiss in not recognizing this fact. Perhaps some day the physician will come to realize that he has a very potent ally at his side who, by her very humanness and tender care, can heal more patients than can a silk suture." The letter ended with the observation that the silk suture and the humanness of physicians and nurses need to be more closely united "before we can look forward to health as we anticipate it."

THE CLINICAL NURSE AS MINISTER TO THE HEALING ART

Implicit in the obstetrician's statement, it is believed, is a function of incomparable importance for the professional nurse of the future who works in the clinical field. Like the physician, she needs proficiency in recognizing the many symptoms of illness and in carrying out complex technical procedures. Much more, however, she needs proficiency in acting as the doctor's ally and colleague in the healing art and in helping patients toward a more positive approach to health. First she must be sensitized to human beings who are sick; she must attempt to understand them by learning to put herself in their place. "How would *I* feel were I little, old Mrs. Jones who has never been a patient in a hospital before and is facing an operation for carcinoma tomorrow morning? What would be going on inside me if I were Mr. Smith about to return after a 'nervous breakdown' to a family of five dependent persons and no job?"

Having developed something of this sensitivity and understanding, the nurse must have time at her disposal for establishing a nurse-patient relationship for which she has already received preparation and through which sympathetic interest, much undisturbed but active listening, and some quiet talking are possible. Only in such a way can she provide the emotional comfort and satisfaction that are basic to the healing art, obtain supplementary facts essential for the planning of further therapy, and informally carry on a teaching function in which reorientation of patient attitudes will probably be as important as instruction in physiology and technical procedures.

Because the writer considers the paragraphs as applicable to the clinical nurse as to the general practitioner of medicine, she wishes to quote the opinion offered by the group of psychiatrists mentioned in the first chapter to those physicians who were being helped to introduce psychotherapeutic elements into their daily practice. Only the word "nurse" need be substituted wherever "doctor" appears.

Sick people are essentially dependent people looking for security, and they find that security primarily in their feelings and attitudes toward you as a doctor. Consequently just being the kind of doctor who understands those feelings and attitudes is tremendously helpful to many sick and troubled and uncertain people. More than that, you give these people an opportunity [to talk]. You do this best when you listen and say as little as possible and permit the patient all the freedom he may need to share his troubles with you, for it is in this talking and sharing that a large part of therapeutic usefulness lies. The patient is relieved of anxiety by the mere fact that for the first time he can talk freely about some things. Most of you have had the experience of having a patient say, "This is the first time that I've really been able to talk freely about this." Don't underrate this as therapy. This is very important therapy. It may seem relatively casual to you, but it is the very crux of therapy. It is an important function you are filling in just doing that.

You will go beyond that in dealing with some individuals and their internal problems. You have already learned that as patients discuss these things you find that they have strange attitudes, misinformed attitudes, that they've been frightened, that they are completely at sea about what their illness means. Part of your job, then, is the explanation of what these things really mean in their lives. This can be very surprising, very new to the patient but it can also be tremendously valuable therapeutically, for in so doing you take all the anxiety and the sting away from the somatic or organic interpretation and put it where it rightfully belongs, in the area of the patient's personality. That very frequently brings an immediate relief.[1]

Difficulties in Extending Psychotherapy

There are many individual nurses who appreciate, as did the members of the workshop and the director of nursing service who has been quoted, how important is the kind of nursing care that seeks to alleviate anxiety and fear, to provide strong emotional

[1] Witmer, Helen L., editor, Teaching Psychotherapeutic Medicine; An Experimental Course for General Physicians. New York, Commonwealth Fund, 1947, p. 212.

support during the severe phases of sickness, and to help the patient during convalescence gradually to regain freedom from dependency. Such nurses see how potentially great are the implications, could they work particularly with prospective mothers and children before sickness and emotional problems develop.

But certain difficulties loom large when those responsible for planning programs of nursing service or of student education attempt to grapple with this concept of nursing care. How is it possible for the institutional nurse to focus attention upon such care when large numbers of prescribed technical procedures and treatments must be carried through? As yet, scarcely any hospitals have succeeded in providing the requisite time—except to private duty nurses, most of whom are totally unprepared to use it for this kind of constructive end. A few nurse administrators and educators have become so alarmed at the present and probable future proportions assumed by technical procedures that they assert that immediate relief must be found through making internes or especially trained technicians responsible for a major part of this burden. Unless this be done, they see subsequent deterioration rather than improvement in those aspects of nursing care that depend upon the use of words and of psychological skills.

Another difficulty visualized by these nurse administrators and educators arises from the supposed reluctance of physicians to entrust nurses, even under medical supervision, with considerable responsibility for participation in psychotherapy. That there has been considerable reluctance cannot be denied. Much of it could be completely justified because of limitations in the professional education and emotional maturity of the individual nurse. Much, however, has been rooted in a less defensible cause of a broadly generic nature. Although marked changes are appearing among the younger doctors and those with larger psychological insight, physicians generally have been conditioned to assume that they alone stand on the pinnacle of knowledge and skill in regard to

86

health matters; that nurses were intended to be their hand-maidens. This unreasoned, frequently unconscious assumption has produced thoughtlessness, wastefulness, and neglect of count-less opportunities for better service to patients.

Can anyone calculate the damage to a more sturdy develop-ment of the nursing profession that has come from that one little symbolic act of men physicians permitting or expecting women nurses to hold doors open for them to pass through? If the reader thinks such matters unimportant, he should see the emotional satisfaction of nurses in a hospital where a particular physician habitually opens the door, turns to the nurse with a charming, playful smile, and says, "After you, my dear," and where another doctor attempts to overtake a nurse with a heavy tray in order to carry it down the corridor for her. Just because doctors have been so badly conditioned that they are often unaware of those who work in closest contact with them *as human beings*, it is not surprising that they have largely overlooked the significant role that nurses might play in psychotherapy.

Physicians too frequently know almost nothing, and have little curiosity to learn, about nursing education unless they happen to lecture in a school of nursing or have been persuaded to serve on a committee of the school. It has rarely occurred to them to discover what preparation is being provided in under-standing the emotional component of disease or the influence of the cultural environment upon sickness. Most of them would be profoundly surprised were they to discover how much has been accomplished in recent years in a limited number of places; that there are possibly a few schools where nursing students are today receiving better orientation in emotional and cultural factors than are medical students in the same university.

So unaware of such developments are most physicians that nurse educators and administrators are reluctant to speak as positively as they rightfully could about the nurse's potential contribution in psychotherapy. They fear that physicians will conclude that they are attempting to usurp functions that belong exclusively to doctors. Already the criticism has come to the writer that, in presenting an argument for a broader role for professional nurses, she is seeking to make "pseudo-doctors" of them. For the very reason that her interest is centered in the health of the public and not in the advancement of the nursing profession except so far as that advancement serves the social welfare, she would like to say something about the desirability of interrelated medical and nursing functions that may possibly appear more objective than if it were to come from nurses.

The cost of medical education is so great and thinking about the supply of doctors needed is still so inflexible, that the number of physicians is sharply limited and the outlook is not bright for a large increase in the near future. Yet at the very moment when there are, for example, no more than 4,000 psychiatrists (of whom perhaps only 1,000 are in private practice) and only about 3,500 private pediatricians, both the health services and the public are entering a period of greater insight into the importance of the emotional aspects of sickness and of the maintenance of health as the goal to be pursued. The teaching and listening processes, as essential but time-consuming parts of therapy and of reconditioning the patient, loom large. Can a small medical profession conceivably carry this load alone? If it cannot, can the nurse, as well as the social worker, be brought into a closer team relationship with the doctor in order that the benefits of this newer practice may be as widely extended as possible?

Again it should be noted that the majority of graduate nurses are not now prepared to work safely or effectively in this area. But it appears that the majority of physicians also will need assistance before they, too, know how to engage safely or effectively in psychotherapy. A recent incident serves to illustrate this point. While the writer was walking the services of a well-known teaching hospital, an interne arrived in the men's medical ward on his evening "rounds." The nurse in charge reported a patient with suicidal tendencies for whom she needed a prescription for a sedative drug. The interne spoke sharply about her thinking the man had suicidal tendencies, and then said, in effect, that he did not hold with those who were always seeing suicides under the bed. Very fortunately for the patient (and for the nurse, who with the assistance of only one orderly had responsibility for 27 other sick persons, including one who was dying) he attempted to jump out of the window in the presence of the interne. The drug was immediately prescribed, and on the following morning the patient was transferred to the psychiatric division where provision for his protection was more adequate. It can only be assumed that the medical school from which this young doctor was graduated had failed to give him the necessary familiarity with manifestations of emotional disturbance. More importantly, it had not succeeded in giving him the intellectual humility essential to the best patient care, to good interpersonal relationships, and to his own professional growth and development.

One such case does not constitute conclusive evidence. It is only suggestive. What can scarcely be disregarded, however, are the indications running through Teaching Psychotherapeutic Medicine of how small is the knowledge of experienced general practitioners, not about neuroses and psychoses, but about the physician-patient relationship as a therapeutic instrumentality. In spite of years of practice, these representative physicians testified to the absolutely invaluable aid they had received during a two-week course in a most basic tool for their work. Even from the written record one is able to witness their amazement as they watched their psychiatrist teachers gain the confidence of a patient, and frequently elicit from him a ready flow of relevant talk that they had earlier had no such success in obtaining.

The average physician would seem to be in much the same position as the nurse in needing instruction in simple methods of psychotherapy. If he can learn such methods, cannot the professional nurse? Is it not possible that in this new dynamic area of

learning experiments should be undertaken in providing orientation to representatives of both groups meeting together? Could
these experiments not also concern themselves with the subsequent "together" roles that physician and nurse might play in
supplementing the efforts of each other?

In a few medical schools visited for the purpose of this study
most promising attempts were under way to prepare resident
doctors for a richer understanding of what lies behind sickness
besides organic disease. Time, energy, enthusiasm, and money
were being poured into the effort. Almost always one or perhaps
several nurses were present at clinical discussions. But they were
there as guests. There had been no planned effort on the part of
the medical school to visualize the valuable contribution it might
make to their preparation for close cooperation with the physician.

The writer asked one distinguished surgeon if he did not feel
that the medical profession could afford to be generous in utilizing some of its exceptionally rich educational resources provided
by society, toward helping to build a sector of nursing that was
truly professional. It was not a matter of generosity, he replied,
it was a matter of *absolute obligation*.

Another difficulty, besides lack of time and uncertainty of
physician attitudes, is encountered by nurse administrators who
attempt to introduce more of the nursing care that has here been
designated as the healing art. It centers in the inadequacy of
many nurses in supervisory positions to understand and foster
this type of care which is new to them, and in the inability of
many clinical nurses to provide such care because of emotional
conflicts within themselves. There are still head nurses, even in
those very hospitals where efforts are being made to broaden the
concept and practice of nursing care, who have been so conditioned by their own educational experience that they believe that
any staff nurse not on her feet and in physical movement is "not
working." In the past the giving of a bed-bath to the patient

afforded opportunity for the establishment of an intimate although brief nurse-patient relationship, and yet satisfied the head nurse that work was going on. Now the bath is coming to be given by a nongraduate nurse, before much provision has been made for other ways in which this important relationship can be established.

So far as the clinical nurse is concerned, considerable maturity of personality development is a prerequisite for this type of nursing care. If she herself is insecure, frustrated, emotionally unsatisfied, tense, punitive, how can she give supportive care to sick persons who have much anxiety and fear? How can she help them to reestablish a more normal emotional balance which she herself does not have? The authoritarian atmosphere pervading many hospitals, to which reference was made earlier, is one of the greatest handicaps to personality development. Nothing short of a revolution in the philosophy and practice of many hospitals and their nursing schools will produce an environment sufficiently free and permissive for the nurse to have an opportunity to grow toward the gentleness, kindness, inner quietness and security, and sensitivity essential for performing the healing art. Given an altered environment, however, and the recognition of the nurse as the physician's colleague in ministering to the total needs of the patient, larger numbers of young women of greater educational and emotional maturity might be attracted to professional nursing. Conceivably these changes might also provide a challenge to men, many more of whom are seriously needed in nursing.

As the writer visited schools and their clinical teaching facilities in various parts of the United States, she gained the impression that nurse administrators and educators had relatively less insight into how tight and restrictive the psychological environment still is than into almost any other problem of nursing education. Although appreciable advances have been made toward greater freedom, with the conditioning these policy-makers have undergone as students, it is difficult for them to see how much more needs to be done. The situation varied greatly from school to school. In some where one least expected it, there was a degree of permissiveness that did much to offset limitations of other kinds. In a few places where much might have been expected, accomplishment may have been considerable in terms of the distance traveled but not in terms of contemporary goals achieved.

Occasionally directors said simply and sincerely that they had lived so exclusively within the hospital system that they had little for comparison that would help them to view where they stood. It has occurred to the writer that the consultative services of a Lawrence K. Frank, who could combine insight into personality development and a friendly objectivity in analyzing the environment, might be of great help to such administrators. They would find the mutual exploration of existing situations no threat. Rather would it be a stimulating intellectual and emotional experience. They, in turn, might be able to interpret the help they had received to other directors less prepared to request formal consultation.

Necessity for Increasing Salaries and Prestige

A final problem of a distinctly different nature faced by nurse administrators is that of holding competent personnel in clinical nursing once they have been obtained. Nursing education has progressed to the point where its leaders have confidence in their ability to plan for the preparation of truly professional persons for clinical practice. But once such persons are graduated, they are almost immediately offered supposedly more desirable positions in supervision, administration, teaching, or public health nursing. Because advancement in salary and prestige moves almost everywhere on a vertical rather than a horizontal plane, clinical nursing is left without power to hold those very women who would enrich its content and make it more comparable in social usefulness to medical clinical practice. This problem will definitely have to be faced if true professionalism is to be built into nursing service at a point below the supervisory level.

Failure to take any large constructive action earlier has resulted partly from the hope that those positions carrying substantial remuneration and prestige would ultimately be filled, and some recruits with professional education would then be available for clinical nursing. It is feared that such a hope is vain. Unless clinical nursing is raised in quality and in recognition to a very marked degree, professional schools are not likely to be sufficiently patronized to improve the current situation. Young women reared in an intellectually sophisticated milieu will probably not enter a profession in large numbers where standards of practice consistently fall short of what they, or their advisers, consider desirable.

It must be assumed, therefore, that hospitals (and also community health agencies) should seek by every means at their disposal to make horizontal progression as attractive as vertical. The setting of several appreciably distinct salary levels for clinical nursing would undoubtedly be advantageous. Advancement from one level to another should depend primarily on type of experience and achievement, not on tenure. The almost microscopic increases, now accorded at designated time intervals, exercise little staying influence over the professional nurse with an opportunity to "move up." Increases based on tenure are also desirable, but salary differentiation sharp enough to indicate recognition of accomplishment is even more important.

The purpose of recommending several levels or grades of clinical nursing is to encourage nurses not only to remain in this field but to develop into specialists in a selected clinical subject. As specialists, they should be expected to engage both in practice and in research, writing, consultation, or clinical teaching. Thus they would come to occupy positions of large responsibility in the care of patients and in the advancement of the health services; they would also occupy positions of prestige in the estimation of their professional colleagues. Were such goals to be achieved, however, the hospital would have to make provision for upper salary brackets in clinical nursing well above the lower brackets in supervision.

Many hospitals will promptly say that no budget could stand such drastic upgrading of salaries. The writer certainly does not claim any competence in matters of budget. It appears, however, that the way the hospital dollar is spent needs reconsideration. Perhaps the total salary item would be less affected than supposed, if proportionately more assistant service were used, on the one hand, and if more efficient professional nursing personnel were used, on the other. Unless salary schedules can be utilized as a far greater instrumentality for incentive than at present, any plans for the preparation of professional clinical nurses seem largely futile.

As the nation moves into an era of new hospital construction, one further consideration must be kept in mind. It will ill become an institution that has spent vast sums on luxurious buildings to fail to pay adequate salaries to its personnel. John M. Glenn, long general director of Russell Sage Foundation and member of the board of trustees of the Johns Hopkins Hospital, was heard on more than one occasion to say that were he building a hospital, he would use the most inexpensive materials that would serve functional purposes. But he would seek to put inside the hospital all the equipment available that would benefit patients, and to staff the institution with the finest personnel, regardless of cost, that could be brought together.

At the end of this long discussion of the professional clinical nurse we recommend *that hospitals attempting to engage in more complex forms of patient care analyze their clinical nursing service, interpersonal relationships, and hospital budgets to determine how: (1) a better balance between present technical nursing procedures and psychotherapeutic nursing care can be established; (2) representatives of the medical, nursing, and social work professions can be brought into closer team relationships for the purpose of extending better psychological care to patients; (3) the hospital environment can be changed to foster the nurse's professional growth; and (4) salaries can be paid competent professional nurses adequate to induce them to remain in the clinical field.*

The Nursing Specialist

The second large area in which the services of professional nurses are absolutely essential is the nursing specialties. At present they comprise supervision, administration, teaching, consultation, planning and promotion of professional activities, and public health nursing at least above first level positions.[1] As was implicit in the preceding section, there are yet almost no specialists in clinical nursing. Even advanced courses offered by universities under the title of clinical specialties are designed primarily for persons who will be head nurses and supervisors. Provision for the development of some specialists within clinical nursing has been viewed in this report as necessary if the base on which nursing service rests is to be strengthened, and if the profession is to look forward to a sound, healthy development.

On the other hand, there is growing consensus that public health nursing should not be considered a specialty so far as first level positions are concerned.[2] Opportunity should certainly be provided, as in clinical nursing, for many staff practitioners to become true specialists. The supervisory, administrative, con-

[1] Only because this brief study does not permit discussion of industrial nursing has it generally been included under the term, "public health nursing." Already this sturdy offshoot from the parent stem is well on the way to mapping out a large and important field of cultivation.

[2] The writer regrets the paucity of space devoted throughout the report to public health nursing: an area of particular interest to her and to all those who are as much concerned with the protection and maintenance of health as with the more limited goal of the cure of sickness. The reason this important specialty has been accorded so little attention is that it represents the sector of nursing where a solution of problems has most nearly been reached. Although much remains to be done in further expansion, improvement, and coordination of services, leadership and a sense of direction are apparent. Hence it has seemed necessary to utilize these few pages chiefly for consideration of the institutional field where problems of large magnitude are particularly pressing.

sultant, and educational personnel would naturally continue to be viewed as specialists. But time and experience have brought changes in thinking about first level positions. Regardless of concerted efforts, it was impossible before the recent war to get nearly enough staff nurses who had had a year's university preparation in public health nursing beyond the basic curriculum. There seems to be no proportionately larger likelihood for the years ahead. Hence nurses with only the basic course have had to be employed in large numbers, and helped through in-service training to some understanding of the philosophy of public health nursing with its emphasis upon preventing and reducing sickness and building positive health, and with the teaching process as an essential skill for achieving these goals.

As collegiate schools of nursing have developed, it has come to be believed that preparation designed for beginning positions in public health nursing can and should be built into the basic curriculum. Thus women would be ready to enter this field upon receiving the baccalaureate degree in nursing. (What is even more important for nursing education as a whole is the growing realization that the broader approaches to the social and health aspects of nursing should be a fundamental part of the training of every nurse regardless of her later field of work.) Consequently four collegiate schools, three of which are within universities, have already developed preparation in public health nursing as part of the basic curriculum to the point where it has received accreditation from the National Organization for Public Health Nursing. Several others have asked or will soon ask for accreditation for similar plans. Some of the hospital schools with larger financial resources and the ability to command resources for field work for their students are also cultivating this area.

Returning to the subject of the nursing specialties in general, it should be said that it is here that those nurses who can thus far be designated as professional are largely concentrated. Even in every one of the specialties there are some who have had neither a college background nor more than their basic training as preparation for the positions they are filling. Organized nursing, however, has made a valiant effort in the face of severe odds to enrich the general education and to enlarge the competence of those nurses who wished to engage in supervision, administration, teaching, planning and consultation, and public health nursing. The enrollments of graduate nurses, sometimes running into many hundreds, in those universities where curricula for R.N.s are offered, attest the success of nursing in emphasizing further preparation and the interest indicated by the individual nurse.

The largest number of specialists is in supervision and administration. Many of them also carry responsibilities for teaching nursing students. What they have accomplished in these fields is nothing short of phenomenal, if one considers not only the educational handicaps encountered, but the fact that nursing supervision and administration have received little of the scientific study and careful consideration accorded comparable specialties in much of industry and business. There the "profit-making motive" has furnished large stimulus to efficiency, which has been lacking in nonprofit enterprises. The small hospital or agency has often become the big institution or organization before management has been sufficiently aware of the growth to make any adequate provision. To a rapid on-going process of development, adjustments have been made as well as possible, almost on a day-by-day basis. The nursing service has been no exception.

Anyone who has sat observantly in the office of the director of nursing service of a five-hundred-bed general hospital, let us say, can scarcely fail to be impressed with the size of the job of operating such a service. The director occupies a position that a well-administered industrial plant or department store would rank very high in salary, prestige, and amount of attached professional and clerical assistance. Rarely has the director of nursing service achieved comparable recognition. The director in one teaching hospital was found not to have the quiet and privacy of an office of her own. Frequently directors and their supervisory personnel, together with the meager secretarial staff provided, were seen crowded into two or three small rooms already overflowing with file cabinets. Large institutions have been visited where the hospital superintendent so little understood what constituted good administration that he thought the nursing director should spend part of each day walking the hospital in a supervisory capacity. Such practices do not make for efficiency of service or for economical management. They are survivals of a past day.

We are moving into an era when it is believed that teaching hospitals must necessarily be large and regional hospitals should have from one hundred to two hundred beds, if professional expertness is to be available. Even in the small community hospitals a greater degree of administrative efficiency is contemplated than has formerly existed. For these reasons the whole task of supervision and administration of nursing service needs to be reevaluated, institution by institution, often with the help of professional consultants. Nurses should be given all the assistance possible in making the transition to still larger responsibilities. Particularly important is it that hospital administrators be able to provide not only suggestive principles for procedure but sympathetic interest and understanding.

When one turns to the other, still very small specialties, he finds a distinct possibility that a fresh and conspicuously enlarged contribution may soon come from many more nurses who find places of great social and professional usefulness in consultation, planning, research, writing, and the promotion of nursing and health services, whether on a local, national, or international scale. That their social vision and their achievement have been so large in the past, in view of the restricted horizons of most nursing education, is the wonder. The fact remains, however, that accomplishment has been exceedingly small in some of these areas when measured by professional standards. Scientific research and writing have been negligible. So have been experimental demonstrations in such matters, for example, as the setting up of prepaid nursing care. Attempts to coordinate their knowledge of the community and their special skills with those of other health groups and social workers for the creation of community health programs are still too few.

But some definitely encouraging signs are to be seen. Administrators of expanding public health programs often expect public health nurses to share responsibility with physicians and other specialists in the development of these programs. As schedules for hospital construction are being drawn on a statewide basis, several official bodies have asked nurses or nursing associations to make over-all surveys of the nursing personnel that would be necessary for greatly increased numbers of beds, and to recommend the kinds of preparation needed by this personnel. Teams of specialists that include a nurse are progressively appearing, particularly in connection with the development of programs sponsored by the United States Public Health Service. In planning for mental hygiene, to give only one illustration, a psychiatric nurse finds herself working with a psychiatrist, a psychiatric social worker, and a clinical psychologist.

The most consequential step probably ever attempted by the nursing profession to prepare for these broader functions is its present effort to substitute for six policy-making associations on the national level either one or two new, better financed and administered, and hence more effective professional associations. It has been a courageous, forward-looking, and in general socially motivated act, well ahead of anything comparable in other professions. The very size and complexity of the task, however, have resulted in various difficulties that still have to be resolved. To the extent that mergers of existing associations can be achieved, the profession will have at its disposal instrumentalities for greatly increased effectiveness.

To end this chapter the writer would like to substitute for recommendations of her own two paragraphs written by Dr. Thomas S. Parran, until recently Surgeon General of the United States Public Health Service, to Miss Hortense Hilbert, formerly chairman of the Joint Committee on the Structure of National Nursing Organizations.

"The demands of the present and future are . . . exacting. Health programs are expanding rapidly. The growing body of new knowledge about health must be applied effectively in action programs. These will involve broad understanding of the needs of the people and of the contribution of all kinds of health workers in meeting these needs. Coordinated study by physicians, health officers, nurses, and all related personnel aimed at formulation of sound programs must accompany action.

"The nursing profession will make its best contribution only when it is organized to work with the public and to find its place in the team of allied professional groups. Its organization must be such as to promote research in nursing itself and in nursing as a part of the over-all health program. It must set up channels through which new ideas can be received, evaluated, and used. It must devise a more effective educational system. It must choose wisely for its immediate action among all the problems which confront it. To choose less focal problems would mean failure of nurses to make the contribution the people and the nation expect of them. Such decisions in these times require the best wisdom available among nurses, the planners of health programs, and consumers of services."

V

EDUCATION FOR PRACTICAL AND GRADUATE BEDSIDE NURSES

THUS far attention has been centered on the probable nature of health and nursing services in the years ahead, and on suggestions for facilitating needed changes in the latter. Only now is it possible to attempt to foresee what general education and technical training will be essential as preparation for future nursing services. If there be validity in the earlier analysis of diversity of nursing functions, it follows that there must be diversity in the kinds of preparation requisite for efficient performance of those functions.

PREPARATION FOR THE PRACTICAL NURSE

In-service training has already been noted as a potentially effective method to prepare persons, whether they be called attendants, nursing aides, or by some other name, to perform the simpler nursing functions under supervision. Nothing more needs to be said here except to repeat that in-service training is an entirely appropriate function for the hospital or health agency to cultivate, but one whose great usefulness has yet received far too little attention.

The question of who should provide training for the practical nurse is not so easily answered. There are at present 58 schools that have been approved by state boards charged with such matters or by the National Association for Practical Nurse Education.[1] They may be roughly classified as of three types. First are

[1] Because this discussion of education for the practical nurse must be brief, the reader who wishes further information is referred to pages 210–267 of The Practical Nurse by Dorothy Deming, New York, Commonwealth Fund, 1947.

the private schools under the control of boards of management or social agencies, which generally assume responsibility for an initial period of about four months of classroom work and demonstration before assigning their students to a selected hospital for some eight months of practice. Such schools are relatively few in number. Some of them have made a distinctive contribution to the preparation of practical nurses, particularly for home nursing. No one would deny that their efforts should continue. Because of the difficulty encountered in financing these schools and in recruiting enough students who can pay even the modest fees, this type of training fails to offer a pattern capable of large expansion.

Second are schools conducted by hospitals, particularly specialized hospitals that rely largely upon nongraduate nursing service. Nearly half of the accredited schools for practical nurses are of this type. Students "live in," and receive full maintenance and generally a small allowance. All their instruction, whether classroom or practice, is conducted within the hospital. This arrangement greatly facilitates integration of program. On the other hand, almost no attempt is made to prepare them for home nursing or other duties outside the institution.

At present many general hospitals are in the process of discussing the advisability of opening such schools, often as a substitute for, or in addition to, their "regular" schools of nursing. Two distinct points of view have been expressed about the wisdom of this undertaking. Some persons maintain that the many hospitals now conducting schools for the training of graduate nurses where clinical facilities and education staffs are inadequate could make a larger contribution to nursing by preparing practical nurses. Others fear that these hospitals generally would not fulfill even this more limited function, because they would still be subjected to pressures that would result in putting nursing service before education. Moreover, they could scarcely be expected to offer training for home nursing, regardless of the fact that the need for practical nurses to care for chronics, convalescents, and

102

subacute illness in homes is desperate. For these reasons such persons believe that the administration of training should be reposed within the public education system, and more specifically within vocational or adult education.

This brings us to the third and newest type of training, the "vocational" curriculum, which sometimes is, and sometimes is not, conducted by a public vocational school. Customarily three months of theory and practice in a nursing arts' laboratory are provided within the school building. Then students are sent for practice with actual patients to a designated hospital. Few of these schools as yet give supervised practice in homes or preparation for other noninstitutional fields. If the curriculum is in a publicly supported school, no tuition is charged to residents of the state. Hospitals, furthermore, usually pay an allowance to students during the practice period.

Although training of practical nurses within public vocational schools is still very far from satisfactory, certain influences are at work which emphasize the probable desirability of placing instruction there and which may greatly improve the curricula offered. A strong inducement is the fact that federal funds are available under the Smith-Hughes and George-Barden Acts (the latter being formerly known as the George-Deen Act) to supplement the salaries of teachers, supervisors, and directors engaged in vocational education. Similarly state funds are often granted to assist local education boards. The large educational facilities and equipment of many vocational schools, in the use of which programs for practical nurses would share, are coming to be viewed as distinctly advantageous.

Attempts to improve the soundness of curricula are several. The concerted promotional efforts of the National Association for Practical Nurse Education; the official pronouncement of the six national associations referred to in an earlier chapter; and a recent generous grant by the Kellogg Foundation for experimental work in Michigan are examples. One of the most significant undertakings has been an activity analysis made by a carefully selected committee and with the sponsorship of the United States Office of Education. Some 300 procedures were identified as wholly or partly within the competence of practical nurses. This two-year study was published in 1947 by the Office of Education under the title, Practical Nursing; An Analysis of the Practical Nurse Occupation with Suggestions for the Organization of Training Programs. Its phenomenally large sale indicates the interest shown in the subject. At present another federally sponsored committee is attempting to build from this analysis a curriculum that can be recommended to schools of practical nursing.

In early discussions with the Professional Advisory Committee an expression of opinion was asked concerning preparation of the practical nurse. The Committee decided unanimously, after long consideration, that training should be provided by vocational or adult education units of the public school system. It recommended that the period of training be one year, divided between classroom and bedside instruction, and that an understanding of the patient as well as nursing techniques be emphasized. It recommended, furthermore, that in order to give the public some assurance of competence the practical nurse be expected to practice for one year under supervision, but on full pay, within a hospital or agency. Only then should she enter private practice in the home or other field where supervision is often negligible.

With much in these recommendations the writer heartily agrees. For the very reason, however, that training of practical nurses has previously tended to be haphazard in conception, organization, and promotion, she is inclined to believe that substantial further experimentation is desirable before any recommendations can wisely be made which would tend to set organizational patterns. Although it appears theoretically desirable that new training schools be placed under educational auspices, vocational high schools still have to prove that they can provide efficient programs, including supervision of the clinical portion and attempted integration of preclinical and clinical work. They must also prove their ability to attract qualified students. Until such demonstrations have been achieved, it would not be wise to close the door to sincere attempts at sound experimentation by privately organized schools or by hospitals.

The Committee's recommendation concerning a year of supervised practice appears excellent. It ought to do much to increase competence to a degree whereby society might be guaranteed some rightful protection. The important fact should not be overlooked that supervised practice could be provided, in the judgment of the Committee, either within a hospital or a nursing agency. We would greatly hope that practice might frequently be, at least in part, within an agency that offers visiting nursing service under careful supervision. Thus the practical nurse would gain experience in dealing with home situations, which would be invaluable should she subsequently engage in private practice in homes or continue as a staff member of a visiting nursing service.

Going beyond what the Professional Advisory Committee was asked to consider, one further statement must be made. *No system of training for practical nurses is likely to succeed unless the public that creates broad general policy and provides funds, educators who design and operate instructional programs, hospitals and agencies that provide clinical facilities, and nursing associations and state boards of control that set standards and influence recruiting are prepared to manifest an* ACTIVE *interest in practical nursing far beyond any interest yet shown.* Weak as has been much of the training of graduate nurses, achievement has been brilliant when compared with accomplishment in this, almost equally important, sector of nursing. Not only the availability of nursing care for large portions of the population, but also the future status of professional nursing itself will be determined by the degree to which rapid and effective action can be achieved in this long-neglected field.

105

The Graduate Bedside Nurse

We come now to the question which is the most difficult of all to discuss. It is the question of whether a graduate bedside nurse similar to many general and private duty nurses of the present would be needed, if successful preparation of practical nurses on the one hand, and of truly professional nurses, on the other, should be achieved. Recent years have seen considerable clarification of those functions for which training of from a month to a year may be sufficient, and equally of those functions which can be efficiently performed only by persons with professional education. The unsolved problem is whether personnel to give nursing care of an intermediate kind will be necessary.

This question has been discussed with the Professional Advisory Committee and with many individual representatives of nursing and other health services. Much of the group discussion at the three regional conferences indirectly revolved around it. Answers given have appeared to be unsatisfactory for several reasons. Often discussants have had difficulty in visualizing a really well-developed system of assistant nursing service and an equally well-developed system of professional nursing service. Unless such systems can be clearly pictured as accomplished ends, any discussion of the probable need for an intermediate type of nursing service is useless. Without such differentiation we shall almost inevitably have to continue to depend on the graduate bedside nurse as we do today, regardless of the fact that her training has been too long and expensive for performing the simpler functions and not nearly substantial enough for handling complex situations.

Another reason discussions have been unsatisfactory is that many persons are unable to consider this question on its own merits. Almost immediately they associate it with their concept of the hospital school, which has heretofore carried the responsibility for the preparation of graduate general nurses. If they

106

have been favorably impressed with this kind of school and its product, they are likely to conclude that such nurses will naturally be needed in the future. If they are antagonists of the system, they will probably maintain stoutly that nursing should be done exclusively by professional nurses and practical nurses, all of whom have been prepared in educational rather than in service institutions.

The most important reason for not obtaining a satisfactory answer is that objective studies are not yet available for formulating an answer. Thus far, as already noted, nursing functions at the left and right extremes of a horizontal line have been rather clearly delineated. It is recognized that certain functions at the left end of the line can be performed efficiently by nongraduate personnel; that other functions at the right end relating to complex clinical practice and the nursing specialties can be performed only by professional nurses. What is not yet known, as far as the writer can discover, is how far toward the middle of the line the two types of personnel can or should move. To what extent will the future practical nurse be able to carry a considerable burden for assisting under supervision with the care of the acutely ill? How far will the truly professional nurse be expected to engage in bedside care of illness which, although acute, may be relatively uncomplicated?

We have seen in the preceding chapter the exacting nature of nursing procedures, to say nothing of possible psychotherapeutic care, in those hospitals that receive patients on referral. Will it ultimately be concluded that all nursing care in such hospitals, which the nongraduate staff cannot handle, should be provided by professional nurses? Or will there continue to be a distinct place on general and private duty for graduate bedside nurses? Is the situation different in community hospitals that receive less complicated cases? Will there be a larger potential role for them in these institutions? Is it possible that further advances in medical and physical sciences will so raise required standards of practice that even the community hospitals will come to demand something comparable to the nursing currently afforded by the teaching hospitals?[1]

These are a few of the unanswered questions that make it impossible now to determine whether continuing arrangements for the preparation of graduate bedside nurses will be requisite or not. Partial answers can and should be found at the earliest moment. Activity analyses are badly needed to show what constitutes current practices in bedside nursing in a variety of situations. Plans for one such activity analysis on a statewide basis are being drawn at present. If it is commissioned and carried through with the best research techniques available, its usefulness should be large. To any extent that its director is able to predict future trends from an examination of current nursing practices, its validity for prolonged reference will be enhanced. One must remember, however, that dynamic forces are working within the health services, including medical schools, nursing schools, and hospitals. Hence changes in the demands made upon nursing are likely to be frequent and profound. Nothing short of a permanent research committee operating on a nationwide basis could provide the continuing factual data essential for formulation of important policy about the staffing of different kinds of hospitals in different sections of the country.

Proposals Concerning Hospital Schools of Nursing

Although no answer can now be given to whether graduate bedside nurses will be needed if and when full development comes to assistant and professional nursing, certain things can

[1] So far as public health nursing is concerned, similar questions do not exist. Because of the relatively large responsibility that every staff nurse is expected to assume, particularly for teaching health, emphasis has consistently been placed on utilizing personnel as nearly professional as possible. The problem with which public health nursing is now engaged is that of the role of the practical nurse within the visiting nursing team.

and must be said about those hospital schools that have almost without exception prepared such nurses.

Whether one approves the system of hospital schools or not, the continued existence of a considerable number is essential for an interim period until adequate other facilities have been established and are sufficiently patronized to guarantee a steady flow of personnel into nursing. At present provisions for the preparation of practical nurses are negligible when compared with what are needed. Nursing curricula in degree-conferring institutions are more readily available, and many collegiate and university schools have potential openings for far more students than are now enrolled in the basic course. If all hospital schools were to terminate their existence this year, however, the consequences would be disastrous.

Socially Undesirable Schools

The foregoing paragraph most emphatically does not indicate that all hospital schools have a mandate to continue. It does not indicate that even one hospital school necessarily has a mandate to continue indefinitely. Evidence presented briefly in a preceding chapter suggests that a great many schools of nursing should be closed immediately. This conclusion is sharpened by the results of the evaluations, made by responsible nurse consultants of the United States Public Health Service, of the 1,125 schools of nursing that participated in the program of the Cadet Nurse Corps. Seventy-six schools were rated *very poor* and 256 *poor*. Thus almost 30 per cent fell below the grade of *fair*, in which category 646 schools were placed. Only 147 schools, or 13 per cent of the total, received a rating of *good* or *excellent*.[1] The writer's examination of the data made available by the federal office convinced her that if the evaluations had erred, it was generally on the side of leniency.

[1] The United States Public Health Service wishes it specifically understood that the rating of individual schools *cannot* be furnished upon request.

There is and has long been wide consensus that an undetermined number of weak schools—running certainly into several hundreds—should be closed. What possible justification, other than procurement of student nursing service, is there for continued operation of inefficient, small units of training? Three hundred schools averaging 300 students each, or 450 averaging 200, would care for 90,000 students. Medical schools, which believe they must limit enrollments sharply, averaged 277 students prior to the war and the figure is now close to 300.

Evidence, moreover, is available to show that existing large schools of nursing tend to operate far better educational programs than do small schools. A table prepared from the evaluations noted above showed that of the 42 schools that had enrollments of 300 or more students, 67 per cent were classified as excellent or good; 31 per cent as fair; and 2 per cent (one school) as poor or very poor. By contrast, of the 602 schools that had fewer than 100 students only 4 per cent were excellent or good; 50 per cent were fair; and 46 per cent were poor or very poor.

In spite of the considerable agreement that weak schools perpetuate an injustice to the student, the patient, and the community at large, most of them continue to function.[1] No amount of logic or reference to the broader public welfare is likely to close more than an occasional school as long as the hospital board finds in this apprenticeship system a readily available and often profitable source of nursing service for its particular institution. Whenever questions are raised, the board simply counters with the statement that it could not staff the hospital without a school. Every informed person is aware that the problem of staffing is a difficult one, but the general difficulty is probably being enhanced instead of mitigated by the continuation of a system of socially undesirable schools. More than 5,000 hospitals

[1] Those persons who assume that poor schools are dying rapidly of attrition will be interested in the following figures. In 1939 the number of schools accredited by state boards of examiners was 1,328; it has been reduced only to approximately 1,250.

exist that do not operate schools and yet succeed, by some means or other, in providing nursing care. If the supply of trained practical nurses is greatly enlarged and if a system of assignment of student nurses under supervision for experience in community and rural hospitals is evolved, much of the problem of these local hospitals should be solved.

If hospital boards will not themselves put an end to unsatisfactory schools, it seems essential that strong external pressure be exerted on those whose schools fall below certain standards, either to effect necessary changes within a designated time or to close their training units. This is supposedly one of the functions of state boards of nurse examiners. Unfortunately the accomplishments have been distinctly disappointing, as members of state boards themselves often declare. Minimum standards in many states have been set below what any objective analysis would pronounce requisite. More consideration has been given to defining standards that would reflect current practices in the particular jurisdiction than to discovering how the accrediting process could be used as an instrumentality for assuring to the student and the public the values of a thoroughly sound training. "Political considerations" have frequently appeared, it is said, both in appointments made to boards and in decisions and rulings issued by boards.

In spite of such weaknesses, which all too often characterize state examining bodies for other professions as well, we believe that nurse boards can be helped to play a more forward-looking, socially useful, and courageous role. At present many generally responsible members of the community such as physicians, clergymen, teachers, lawyers, club women, and business men, are either entirely apathetic or are found lending their prestige and support to individual hospital schools of inferior quality. If they would exercise some leadership in this matter, the effect upon state boards would be electric. Similarly, if organized nursing would make a substantial examination of all schools in the

111

United States and would then publish an official list of schools it had accredited as competent to meet certain designated educational goals, many state boards would be likely to give prompt attention to revision of their lists.

More effective and immediate action is needed, however, than can be obtained from state accrediting bodies. Hence many thoughtful persons are convinced that either the entire nursing profession moving through existing national associations, or nursing education working through an agency created expressly for the purpose, should throw its weight into the struggle against weak schools. Although repeated studies have emphasized the urgency for closing socially undesirable training units, nursing has never set up accrediting machinery that would bring emphatic pressure on these schools.

Since 1939 the National League of Nursing Education has engaged in careful examination of schools, whether hospital or collegiate, that voluntarily requested accreditation.[1] The process is long and expensive. For a variety of reasons some excellent schools that undoubtedly could qualify for accreditation have not sought it. As a consequence only 110 schools offering the basic curriculum and nine offering affiliation to students from other schools appear on the 1948 list of accredited schools. The process of accreditation is unquestionably of distinct value to many of the schools examined, in providing them with a more objective analysis of their strengths and weaknesses. The published list has considerable usefulness for prospective students and their advisers, but its lack of annotation sharply restricts its usefulness particularly for lay persons in policy-making positions. The purpose of this undertaking is to help relatively good schools to improve and to gain public recognition, and thus indirectly to raise standards of nursing education. It does absolutely nothing to reach schools that were evaluated as very poor or poor and

[1] Several other bodies representing specialized interests in nursing education also engage directly or indirectly in accreditation.

most of those ranked fair by the administrators of the program of the Cadet Nurse Corps.

Subsequent to the close of the war two attempts have been made to reexamine accreditation from a broader base: one by the Committee of Interests in Accreditation, composed of representatives of several national nursing associations, with the counsel of Dr. George A. Works, who has had long experience in accreditation[1]; the other by Raymond Rich Associates, whose "Report on the Structure of Organized Nursing" emphasized particularly the importance of accreditation.[2] Two somewhat different purposes and distinctly different methods of accreditation emerged from these examinations.

The Committee of Interests recommended that there be created an organization of schools of nursing, one of the principal functions of which should be to accredit schools voluntarily applying for membership. It visualized three classes of members: schools offering the basic curriculum, schools offering advanced curricula, and schools preparing practical nurses. This organization would supposedly be the *only* accrediting agency in the field of nursing education. Thus the Committee attempted both to end previous duplication of effort, and to establish enough prestige within a single body to stimulate wider interest among the schools in seeking accreditation. For the membership of the association it outlined a variety of excellent services designed to improve nursing education.

The one weakness of the Committee's plan, in the opinion of the writer, lay in proposed reliance upon voluntary application for membership. It is obvious that hundreds of weak schools would not apply and pay the suggested examination fee, when

[1] Two articles by Mary C. Connor, R.N., "Accreditation—Stimulant or Narcotic?" and "Accrediting and the Structure Study," in the American Journal of Nursing, July and October 1947, respectively, give an excellent statement of the general philosophy behind the work of this committee.

[2] The entire Report was published in the American Journal of Nursing, October 1946, pp. 648–661. Discussion of accreditation appears on p. 659.

they knew that they could not gain membership unless some device such as that used by the American Library Association were employed. For the purpose of accreditation, the ALA prepared minimum requirements for schools on four levels, and then, following examination, assigned each existing school to one of the four levels. Provision was made for inclusion of schools operated by service institutions which it believed should be eliminated. These schools were put in the lowest category. Once they had been brought inside an organizational structure, requirements could be gradually raised, the Association maintained, until they had either closed or had improved sufficiently to be transferred to the next higher level. Within seven years change had been so pronounced that the lowest category was dropped entirely. But the number of schools placed there originally, although larger than in any other group, had been eight. The Association had the task of concerning itself only with a total at that time of 18 schools. Even so, it did not depend upon voluntary solicitation of schools. Nursing has the stupendous job of 1,250 schools to face.[1]

In contrast to the proposal of the Committee on Interests, the Rich Associates argued that accreditation is an almost inescapable responsibility that should be accepted by organized nursing as a whole and should not be delegated. Therefore they recommended that the function be placed within the over-all membership association, and that the full power of that association be rallied behind the process. They insisted that examination of all schools be mandatory. Once criteria for accreditation had been formulated and officially adopted, examination of every existing school should proceed as rapidly as possible, and the list of approved schools should be published.

The "Rich Report" considered it feasible that at the beginning minimum rather than optimum criteria for accreditation should

---

[1] For a more detailed statement of this device, see The Use of Research by Professional Associations in Determining Program and Policy by Esther Lucile Brown, New York, Russell Sage Foundation, 1946.

be used. Thus the number of institutions eligible for approval and hence for automatic membership in a Conference of Accredited Schools of Nursing would be appreciably enlarged. All included could then be constructively helped to further improvement. The Report recommended that organized nursing give the fullest possible measure of support to schools receiving approval, to include not only educational counseling but assistance in recruiting students, placing graduates, and so on. It maintained that conversely support should be withheld from schools failing to meet the criteria for accreditation.

Finally, the Rich Associates made the important suggestion that *since the purpose of accreditation is not primarily to serve the interests of the schools but to serve the public interest and to improve the practice of the profession, no fee should be charged.* "This is inevitably a costly process. But its importance should ensure the full support of organized nursing, the majority of nursing schools, many government and voluntary health agencies, the foundations and the public."[1]

Whatever plan be used, strong and concerted action will be requisite if accreditation is to serve as a form of social control exercised in the public interest. Only a determined struggle, such as that in which Dr. Abraham Flexner and the Council on Medical Education and Hospitals engaged nearly four decades ago in producing a housecleaning of medical schools, is likely to be effective. Twice, extensive nursing school data of inestimable value to the public and the nursing profession have been gathered: during the late 1920's by the Committee on the Grading of Nursing Schools, and again during the recent war by the Division of Nursing of the United States Public Health Service. These data, however, were utilized almost exclusively for counseling purposes. The Committee on Grading mailed confidential reports to each school, rating its position relative to other schools in regard to long lists of items. The Division of Nursing gave the

[1] American Journal of Nursing, October 1946, p. 659.

115

most effective field assistance possible to individual schools participating in the program of the Cadet Nurse Corps. In neither instance was society nor even the nursing profession provided with lists of schools that could or could not meet certain criteria.

Such gentleness will do little to end a disgraceful situation in nursing education. The late Dr. William Cherin, a truly devoted friend to nursing, often remarked, "Nurses have got to learn that there are times when it does not pay to be ladylike. They will have to take their gloves off and fight."

We recommend that nursing make one of its first matters of important business the long overdue official examination of every school; that the lists of accredited schools be published and distributed as far as possible to every town and city of the United States as an avowed substitute (except legally) for the inadequate lists of schools accredited by state boards of nurse examiners; that an unequivocal statement be included in the published document to the effect that any school not named had failed to meet minimum requirements for accreditation or had refused to permit examination; that a nationwide educational campaign be conducted for the purpose of rallying broad public support for accredited schools, and for subjecting slow moving state boards and nonaccredited schools to strong social pressure.

We recommend, further, that provision be made for periodic reexamination of all schools listed or others requesting it, as well as for first examination of new schools, and for publication and distribution of the revised lists.

Finally, we recommend that, if organized nursing commits itself to this undertaking of major social significance, the public assume responsibility for a substantial part of the financial burden.

Relatively Good Schools

Attention must now be turned to those hospital schools where classroom, laboratory, and clinical facilities and teaching personnel are reasonably adequate for sound preparation, at least of a traditional nature, for general bedside nursing. Included in this category would be a considerable proportion of those schools designated as fair and good by the Division of Nursing. Excluded would be those relatively few hospital schools which are most nearly professional in educational program and whose graduates quickly move into complex clinical nursing or into supervisory and administrative positions. They will receive consideration in the next section.

Most schools in this intermediate category have never sought to be professional in the Flexnerian meaning of that term, although some have established relations, often of a tenuous and far from satisfactory nature, with degree-conferring institutions. If it is found that the graduate bedside nurse is eventually not needed, there will be no justification for the continued existence of these schools. Even should she be required, it is probable that nonservice institutions, such as central schools and junior colleges, should assume responsibility for administering this kind of nursing education and for assigning students for part of their clinical experience to many of the hospitals that are now operating these schools.

The fact that the ultimate future of the relatively good hospital schools is uncertain does not absolve them from offering students the best possible preparation for skilled bedside nursing and for familiarity with the general problems of a complete health service. Indeed if these schools would think of themselves as being in a transitional phase, the resulting flexibility in outlook could be utilized as an important aid in the process of improvement. It might even put some of them in a position to be brought finally within a university professional curriculum, should that become desirable.

Improvements, it is agreed, can and *should* be made in most of these schools on many fronts. They need teaching in line with the best contemporary principles of education; more types of clinical experience; better integration of the preclinical and clinical portions of the curriculum; permeation of the entire curriculum with the preventive as well as the curative, and the mental as well as the physical, aspects of nursing; more emphasis upon the care of the ill in the home and in emergency situations; greater attention to the student's physical, emotional, intellectual, and social development; larger consideration of the function of the nurse as a citizen and as a member of the health services.

One fortuitous circumstance growing out of the recent war has been exceptionally valuable in helping these hospital schools to visualize perhaps more clearly than before how some of the needed improvements might be made. Under the exigency of the requirement by the Cadet Nurse Corps that the basic curriculum be completed in thirty months, many schools discovered to their surprise that they could cover adequately in this shorter period instruction of the kind they had been giving. This discovery has led to some fertile thinking about its implications. Should the period of training actually be shortened? Or should the last six months be devoted to selected nursing practice in a particular field? Or should the additional time be used to permit appreciable enrichment of the entire curriculum? If so, should the enrichment be provided by the hospital school or by an institution whose sole function is education?

Much discussion of all these questions is current and a few experiments have actually been instituted. The proponents of a shortened period of study think that it would be possible, with wise planning and adequate resources, to achieve in perhaps little more than two years as much or more than the average reasonably good school achieved in three years prior to the war.[1]

[1] Interestingly enough the Report of the Working Party on the Recruitment and Training of Nurses (London, His Majesty's Stationery Office, 1947, p. 49) takes exactly this position. Training has been unnecessarily long in Great Britain, it maintains, because of the domestic duties and the noneducational nursing service required of students. It recommends a basic course of two years, the first eighteen months of which would be devoted to fundamentals common to all fields of nursing and the remaining six months to concentrated training in one selected field. Provisional state registration would then follow successful completion of an official examination. A third year devoted to salaried nursing practice under supervision would be required before a license was granted permitting the nurse to engage in private practice.

This assumption rests, however, upon the condition that the school devote its entire time to education and be freed of responsibility for nursing service. So convinced are some that almost a year might be saved if education were the exclusive goal, that one distinguished hospital school is about to institute a curriculum of twenty-eight months, and several other schools are considering similar plans.

At the beginning of 1948 an independent demonstration school was opened in Windsor, Ontario, under the sponsorship of the Canadian Nurses' Association and with the financial assistance of the Canadian Red Cross Society.[1] The curriculum has been planned to require only twenty-five months including vacations; the school states, however, that one or two additional months may be necessary. It believes that it can not only cover but make more meaningful the material usually taught in the traditional preclinical and clinical subjects, and can also offer a month's experience in communicable diseases, another month in public health and community nursing, and orientation in mental hygiene and psychiatry and in ward management. The principal clinical laboratory will be the Windsor Metropolitan Hospital, but affiliations are being arranged with other hospitals and the public health field.

The concept of selected nursing practice appears to be winning favor.[2] The six months of service required by the Cadet Nurse Corps and interpreted by it to mean supervised practice, suggested to many that a similar period of time might be used advantageously either to give the student greater proficiency in a particular field of nursing, or to give her experience in a different environmental setting. Some educational directors are of the

[1] As of January 1946 only 13 schools in the United States, out of a total of 1,214 reporting to the National League of Nursing Education, stated that they were independent. Twelve had been separately incorporated and one expected to be.

[2] The word "internship" is sometimes used for this type of nursing practice. It should not be confused with that more advanced kind of internship, which is also being much discussed and is already being utilized to a limited extent as preparation for the nurse with a university degree, who wishes to become a consultant in a field such as orthopedics or mental hygiene.

same opinion as the British Working Party that if a student were to concentrate upon one field of nursing of her choice, she would not only acquire appreciable skill and understanding in the application of basic principles, but the chances would be great that she would wish to continue in that field as a graduate nurse. Other nurse educators consider experience under totally different circumstances more important than a field of concentration. They argue plausibly that training should begin in a large hospital where clinical resources and teaching personnel are rich. But they advocate further that such training be followed by experience in community and rural hospitals where students would have opportunity to see the particular problems encountered by those health services, and where the relationship between the family and community and the individual's health or sickness might be thrown into sharper relief.

Enrichment of the curriculum is understandably one of the means much discussed at present for utilizing the customary thirty-six months of training constructively. Through it many educational directors see a way to achieve those improvements indicated earlier as generally needed. Hence plans are being made to integrate within the course of study more of the social and health aspects of nursing; to give greater attention to the individual student's development; to present some wider picture of the health services as they exist outside the hospital.

Every attempt at enrichment of the curriculum merits the utmost consideration. Current experiments should be multiplied many times. Large numbers of the reasonably good hospital schools are so stereotyped in their program and so lacking in any dynamic quality that such attempts are urgently needed if only to restore their vitality. One important question, however, must be raised. Should enrichment of the curriculum of these schools be undertaken at the expense of prolonging the course even to the customary thirty-six months? In the next chapter the writer will argue that broadening and deepening of the *professional* curriculum are absolute essentials for the preparation for diversity of function and degree of responsibility that professional nurses must assume. In the case of the graduate general nurse, however, emphasis needs to be placed only on preparation for bedside care and some understanding of what constitutes a complete health service. It is not her task to engage in those forms of community nursing where teaching of groups of persons plays an important role, or to undertake the practice of the nursing specialties. Hence the problem seems to be that of defining what kind of program can be included within the framework of a curriculum, preferably shorter than thirty-six months, that will most directly benefit her.

Two instrumentalities have made their appearance that are of signal potential importance in improving the training of the graduate bedside nurse: the central school and the junior college. The writer arranged expressly to visit a central school. It proved to be one that has been assiduously cultivated since its creation in 1932. In the state where this school is situated a religious order of Catholic Sisters conducts three general hospitals. One of 200 beds serves patients on a relatively high financial and educational level who frequently come from long distances to obtain specialized medical care; another, of the same size, serves a highly industrialized and trading center; the third, of 75 beds, is in a mining region where economic and educational levels are exceedingly low, a large proportion of the dominant minority group cannot speak English, and public health statistics still show an appalling picture of maternal and infant mortality and communicable diseases.

Prior to the creation of an independent central school controlled by its own board of directors, the Sisters had operated schools that they knew to be unsatisfactory in these three hospitals. Now all students are matriculated in the central school, where they are provided preclinical training on a much higher level than was previously possible. Thereafter the school arranges for coordinated clinical experience in each of the three hospitals, thus giving the students an opportunity to care for patients widely diversified as to disease and to economic and educational background. Equally good opportunities are available for clinical experience in surgery, medicine, and obstetrics in the two larger hospitals. One has a well-organized pediatric department to which all students are assigned for three months; the other has a nationally known tuberculosis service that is used for a similar period of required training; the hospital in the mining region provides three months of experience, particularly in emergency and first-aid nursing.

Three affiliations with other hospitals or agencies are maintained. One affiliation of three months is in psychiatric nursing either in the psychiatric division of the state general hospital or in the state hospital for the mentally ill, both of whose teaching resources are supervised by the state university. A second, of six weeks, is in communicable diseases in a children's hospital. The third, which is elective, is six weeks of public health nursing in an undistinguished county health unit. At the time of the writer's visit to the school, the Sister Director was arranging for consultative assistance in an attempt to strengthen the public health aspects of the curriculum. The fact that the state has recently embarked on a much enlarged program of public health may ultimately make improved teaching resources available to the school.

Two affiliations are also maintained with academic institutions, a college situated in a nearby city and Catholic University of America in Washington, D. C. Thus students of outstanding ability who complete two and a half years of coordinated collegiate subjects in the liberal arts, either preceding or following the nursing course, may receive the degree of Bachelor of Science in Nursing and thereby pass into the ranks of professional nurses. As in most other places where a similar arrangement has been supplied, relatively few students have availed themselves of this opportunity.

At present initial steps are being taken toward making this school an integral part of a collegiate institution. Although its accomplishments have been so outstanding in comparison with those of its immediate forebears that it provides a pattern for similar undertakings elsewhere, the Sister Director believes that the time is fast arriving when a truly professional school operated by an academic institution and requiring a substantial amount of collegiate general education should be established.

Anyone who witnesses the potentialities inherent in the central school, immediately wonders why the concept has not been translated into action in many scores of instances. Catholic Sisters are reported to operate eight central schools that have replaced 23 former hospital schools. The fact that religious orders administer such large numbers of hospitals and close to 30 per cent of all schools of nursing should facilitate the use of this educational device by them, particularly if cooperation among the various orders is satisfactorily established. But it is an instrumentality, only now beginning to be cultivated, that is admirably suited to nonsectarian as well as sectarian groups.[1] In many compact communities anywhere from two to a dozen hospital schools within a few miles of one another continue to exist as small, mediocre, and isolated teaching units.

One prosperous city of approximately 300,000 population has, for example, six schools not affiliated with a college or university. In January 1948 enrollments ranged from 15 to 129 with an average of 65. One of two facts is almost certain. Either the preclinical and clinical instruction in these six schools is much poorer than need be, or the cost of maintaining adequate instruction is much higher than necessary. Why should these schools not pool their financial resources and their clinical facilities for teaching purposes? Even if one or two of the schools did

[1] For a fuller discussion than is possible here of the central school and particularly of the role of the college in offering centralized teaching, see "The College and Centralization of Nursing Instruction" by Eugenia K. Spalding, American Journal of Nursing, February 1943, pp. 195–201.

not wish to join the plan, a central school serving the educational interests of some four hospitals could unquestionably afford better teaching, particularly in the social sciences and the less cultivated fields, than is provided at present. The budget would allow more numerous and competent clinical instructors than these hospitals can now provide. Probably through rearranged assignment of students the adequacy of clinical facilities could also be enhanced.

The entire tone of nursing education could be raised from its present uninspired level in large numbers of communities through an effort such as this. An important first step would be taken which might make a second step appreciably easier, whether that second step were the incorporation of an independent central school or integration within a junior or other college. Aloofness from the educational world that exists outside hospital walls and persistent clinging to old vested interests are taking a toll of nursing education that can ill be afforded. Unless these hospital schools that we have designated as relatively good can find their future within a larger frame of reference, they are likely to go the way of those socially undesirable schools for which little but extinction remains.

The other significant instrumentality that has demonstrated its value to the hospital school is the junior college. In the state where the public junior college movement has probably had its most conspicuous development as yet, the writer saw in turn a public general hospital of 3,600 beds and a "de luxe" voluntary hospital of 285 beds, both using to their satisfaction the instructors provided by the junior colleges of their respective cities. On the basis of contractual arrangements, these educational institutions sent accredited teachers in the physical, biological, and social sciences directly to the hospitals to conduct courses at no expense either to the hospital or student. The superintendent of schools and the principal of the junior college in one of the cities have stated officially that they considered these semiprofessional courses, offered through cooperative arrangements with local hospitals, one of the most important developments for the junior colleges.[1] The directors of both schools visited assured the writer that the teaching was a marked improvement over what had formerly been provided by the school, and an opportunity had been given for the introduction of courses for which the directors themselves would have had great difficulty in finding instructors.

Can the potential value of such arrangements be overestimated? Now that junior colleges are in process of being created in many states, it might be assumed that organized nursing and hospitals operating schools would become ardent proponents for the development of such colleges strategically located to meet their needs.

In a small city of the state referred to above, one junior college was found which had actually operated a three-year school of nursing since 1945 as an integral part of its program. Science courses offered to student nurses were taught by members of the college faculty who had specialized in those subjects. The educational director of nursing had been associated with a university school that has long emphasized the social and health aspects of the nurse's function. Hence she made provision in the curriculum for far more work in the social sciences and their application than the average hospital school supplies.

During the first semester courses on the maintenance of health in the community and in the family were required prior to the initial course on remedial nursing. Psychology extended over four semesters. The course in the third semester was devoted to mental hygiene, the fourth to child psychology. Social institutions, a study of contemporary society, received two semesters of attention. This course led to a brief survey of community agencies, and a thirty-two-hour examination largely by field observation of the nature of social casework. In the third year elements of public

---

[1] Sexson, John A. and John W. Harbeson, The New American College. New York, Harper and Bros., 1946, p. 269.

health nursing was followed by sixteen hours of principles and practice in health teaching and a similar number in home nursing.

A good county hospital of 430 beds two miles from the college provided the laboratory for clinical instruction. The hospital comprised 170 beds in the acute division, 150 beds in the chronic division, a tuberculosis sanatorium of 110 beds, and an emergency service. A county public health unit maintained offices in a wing of the main building. Except for the chronic division which was to be rebuilt and only then could be opened for teaching purposes, the physical facilities and equipment were excellent. Blueprints and memoranda had already been prepared for further large expansion of the physical plant and for the taking of various health services directly to the outlying rural community. The hospital was staffed by a full quota of resident physicians and by an impressive number of graduate nurses on general duty, as well as in supervisory and administrative positions. One of the most modern and attractive nurses' residences in the United States had been recently completed in a truly beautiful spot only a stone's throw from the hospital.

The remarkable achievements of this school in the brief period since its inception are largely the result: of the phenomenal efforts of the director of nursing service to create the best possible clinical laboratory for the junior college students; of the broad concept of nursing as a community health service which the educational director brought to the college; and of the large degree of cooperation manifested by the board and the administrative officers of the college and by others interested in this community undertaking.

What the ultimate success of the school is likely to be cannot be known for some years to come. There are still many unsolved problems. The economic relations between the hospital and the college, which had not been put on a sound basis in the estimation of the director of nursing service, are now being reconsidered and the hospital will guarantee by written contract to pay for the services of nursing students. A science instructor reported that he had not yet found what subject matter could be given most usefully and expeditiously in courses he considered too short for student nurses who seemed intellectually immature to him. The writer questioned whether the school was not attempting a more ambitious program than could be carried to maximum success in three years. Its broad orientation toward community nursing was primarily professional, but the time devoted to it was less than the university school would deem absolutely essential. This problem will probably be solved through extending the curriculum before long to four years in order to give students more time for intellectual and emotional growth, and better fit them for a rich contribution to community nursing in the area. However that may be, the school is of wide significance as a demonstration of nursing education administered by a junior college, and equally of a wholehearted experiment in enrichment of the curriculum in a nondegree program.

In the light of current needs for graduate bedside nurses and current opportunities for their education, *we recommend that those hospital schools here designated as relatively good make concerted effort through various types of experimentation to increase their vitality and social usefulness and to point the way to an ultimate solution of the "hospital school problem." Experiments in simultaneously shortening the period of training but improving the course of study are particularly needed. Scientifically controlled tests of the educational value of nursing practice in selected areas of concentration and in diverse environmental situations merit initiation. Especially recommended as transitional steps toward the future are the creation of central schools of nursing, and utilization of the teaching resources of junior colleges.*

Distinguished Hospital Schools

Of those schools of nursing which have had a long and distinguished history in providing much of the potential leadership

127

of the profession, some have found a place for themselves as supposedly integral parts of universities. (Unfortunately the organizational structure is often not yet so clear cut as many persons believe desirable, if these schools are to develop to their maximum capacity in the shortest time.) Thus they have become degree-conferring schools and are entitled to the use of the term "professional," exactly as are schools of engineering, law, medicine, theology, social work, business administration, journalism, and so on, that now exist within institutions of higher learning. These university schools are the subject of discussion in the following chapter.

Other schools that have had an equally successful past are still under the control of hospital boards just as they always have been. During the past two decades, however, many of them, like some of the only relatively good hospital schools, have established affiliations with colleges and universities which are willing to credit their basic curriculum with varying numbers of points toward an academic degree.[1] Thus it is possible for their students to receive not only the diploma from a school of nursing but a bachelor's degree by spending usually about two additional years in academic study prior, preferably, or subsequent to the nursing course. The many detailed differences in contractual arrangements entered into between hospital and college or university need not be enumerated here. They have been determined by the official policy of the particular educational institution and the particular hospital school, within the framework of the general philosophy of nursing education current at the time the specific plan was evolved. Most of these "combined programs," however, have produced what is generally known as "the five-year course."

Great hope was reposed in this type of affiliation during its early period. The leading hospital schools which had embarked on these combined programs assumed that so many students

---

[1] In 1946 a total of 91 hospital-controlled schools had some sort of arrangement with a college or university whereby students might receive degrees.

would take advantage of this opportunity that they would be able to raise their course of study to intellectually more mature levels and enlarge the potential leadership of their graduates. This hope has not been realized.

By virtue of the prestige of these schools considerable direct and indirect selection of students is possible. Whether a combined program has been arranged or not, some schools require one year of college work for admission, some two, one briefly required a complete college course. In general, however, high-school graduation has continued to be the only possible compulsory educational requirement. Beyond that, these schools have selected individual applicants with the most diverse educational background who had other needed qualifications such as health, outgoing personality, alertness.

Relatively few of these students have exhibited an interest in obtaining a degree under the combined program. Even where the number of annual graduates is large, those receiving recognition from an affiliated college or university could often be counted on the fingers of two hands.[1] This failure is part and parcel of that depressing saga of a profession where sights have not been lifted because education has almost always had to take second place. What would cause the eyes of the average student nurse to be focused on higher education in a hospital setting where only one curriculum was provided for young women with widely varied amounts of schooling and with the largest numbers in the lower educational categories; where attention, no matter how much the

[1] Nothing makes more dreary reading than a comparison, page after page, of the statistics published by the National League of Nursing Education for total number of students in the basic degree program versus the number enrolled in individual hospital (and *even university*) schools that have made provision for the conferring of degrees. In 1947 no fewer than 40,744 students were graduated from all state-accredited schools of nursing in the United States. Exactly 1,779, or 4 per cent, of this enormous number were reported to have received either a bachelor's or master's degree for the basic course of study. These 1,779 came from 102 schools: 1,327 were from schools operated by colleges or universities, and 45 were from schools controlled both by an institution of higher learning and a hospital. Only 26 of *all* hospital-controlled schools reported graduation of students with degrees; the total number of such students was 407.

director of nursing service and nursing education might regret it, was by necessity chiefly pinned to the daily practice of bedside nursing techniques and not to the continuous examination of the scientific and social base that underlies or might underlie this health service?

Not only has the combined course failed to achieve what had been greatly desired, but these particular hospital schools are discovering that their former preeminent position is becoming threatened by the development of university-operated schools of nursing. Many a girl who is uninterested in what she thinks of as a hospital course and a degree program totaling five years, the administrative details of which seem very complicated and unattractive to her, can be interested in a four-year integrated program offered by a university with its wealth of cultural and social advantages and with its very different outlook on education. The prospects are large that as these university schools grow in number, excellence, and recognition, students will seek them rather than even the three-year course of distinguished hospital schools. Already a few university curricula have been sufficiently successful to cause the leading hospital schools to look upon them as serious potential competitors.

There seem therefore to be two choices for selection by those schools that long furnished the only distinctive basic courses that existed and that still attempt to provide basic training second to none. Before long either they will have to drop into the ranks of semiprofessional schools, or they will have to become integral parts of universities whose avowed goal is professional education. About which choice is socially preferable, there is little question. They belong within the university. Their vast clinical facilities alone are of the kind and complexity that should be at the service primarily of professional and not semiprofessional education. Their orientation toward preparing students for professional clinical practice, as well as laying a base for the nursing specialties, ought not to be lost at the very time when qualitative needs

130

are beginning to be generally understood as truly important. Unless these schools find themselves soon within institutions of higher learning, however, their contribution to the public welfare is likely to be greatly weakened.

Their situation today is comparable to that which Pratt Institute faced a decade ago. Over a long period Pratt had conferred a diploma on librarians, home economists, engineers, art teachers, and architects, whose professional services were greatly demanded everywhere, so outstanding was the preparation afforded by that institution. But degree-conferring universities were in the meantime building curricula in all these specialized areas. The day came when Pratt realized that its whole future was endangered. It would not continue to attract students of first-rate ability or in sufficient numbers unless they knew that they would receive a degree upon completion of the curriculum.

The pressure of educational events forced Pratt, against its will, to take the step of becoming a degree-conferring institution. By so doing it provided for the continuation of outstanding curricula, which had been professional—as of their time—in all but the recognition conferred.

In recent years much planning and money have been expended on weaving considerable amounts of the liberal arts within Pratt's professional curricula. The task is far from complete. If a dynamic institution is maintained, it will never be finished. Increasingly it is being realized everywhere that no technical training, however good, is sufficient as preparation for professional personnel. A broad understanding of the physical and social sciences on which professional practice is built and of the society which the professions serve is essential. Most professional schools that were not parts of universities, however, would probably be less fortunate than Pratt in having the money and the ability to obtain the highly trained teaching personnel required to move into these educational areas that have come to constitute a significant part of professional preparation.

The distinguished hospital schools are faced with this very dilemma. As long as professional training was modest in its demands upon budget, teaching staff, and equipment, these schools could certainly provide the best there was to give. But the prerequisites of contemporary professional education have grown to such proportions that no hospital should endeavor to bear this burden unless its school be heavily endowed, any more than it should bear the burden of conducting a medical school. Only the university can provide from its wealth of available resources what is necessary. For this reason, besides its inability to grant the degree, the longer the distinguished hospital school stays outside the university the less favorable will its position probably be.

So important is it that this transition be achieved and at the earliest possible moment that *we recommend not only that there be expressed conviction that provision should be made within the university for the continuing undiminished contribution of distinguished hospital schools; but that they be given wholehearted assistance in achieving this reorganization by the entire nursing profession, medical and hospital associations concerned with nursing, university and hospital administrators, university faculties, administrators and faculties of schools of medicine and public health, foundations, and those members of the laity influential in effecting policy and influencing public opinion.*

Schools of Specialized Hospitals

Some brief reference must be made to a final category of hospital schools: those operated by specialized hospitals. At present there are 35 such state-accredited schools of which 28 are in hospitals for the mentally ill. With the exception of one federal and two privately operated hospitals, all of the 28 schools are in state hospitals. Although the writer was primarily concerned with the basic curriculum as offered by the general hospital or institution of higher learning, she visited one state hospital of more than 6,000 beds and an even larger federal hospital for the mentally ill, both of which provide basic curricula. In connection with much earlier studies she had visited other schools in state hospitals in many parts of the United States. No school in a public hospital for the mentally ill that she has ever seen was nearly satisfactory either in her judgment or that of the persons administering it.[1] Some were appreciably better than others. They were maintained almost solely because they provided at least a modicum of nursing service more skilled than that attendants could supply.

The problems with which these schools are faced are almost innumerable. In part because of nurses' lack of training for and interest in mental disease, and in part because many of these enormous, drab hospitals are situated in seemingly remote places and have inadequate salary scales, sufficient administrative, teaching, and supervisory personnel can rarely be obtained to staff a school properly or to provide desirable nursing situations for clinical training. Even such limited personnel as is available consists primarily of graduate nurses who have had only limited preparation for work in the psychiatric field. Specialized psychiatric nurses, desperately needed not only for the successful direction of nursing service and nursing education but for the care of patients, are negligible in number.[2] Proportionately the medical staff is no larger or better prepared than the nursing staff. The paucity of psychiatrists in the majority of these hospitals precludes the amount and quality of educational help needed from physicians.

Although these hospitals customarily pay students a monthly stipend (usually of $30) beginning with matriculation, almost all

---

[1] One school that has existed for more than sixty-five years and is operated by a voluntary hospital enjoys a considerable degree of distinction. Unfortunately the writer has not seen it.

[2] An initial report prepared by a Subcommittee on Psychiatric Nursing [in Public Mental Hospitals] for the Hospital Committee of the Group for Advancement of Psychiatry describes the role that the specialized psychiatric nurse could play in these hospitals. The thinking of this subcommittee is so forward-looking that it is hoped the report will be published and widely examined.

are unable to attract enough students to justify any large expenditure for educational purposes. In January 1948 there were 725 students, 217 of whom were men, enrolled in the 28 schools. Half of the schools had from 2 to 21 students. Except for one school of 70, none exceeded 54 students. Even the widely known school just referred to in a footnote had an enrollment of only 25 women and 23 men.

Among the diversity of problems encountered perhaps the most critical is that of providing a sound and varied basic curriculum within a specialized hospital. Following the preclinical classroom period, students are given a period of clinical experience on the medical and surgical wards and in the operating rooms of what is designated as the infirmary or "general hospital." Afterward they are sent elsewhere to general hospitals, usually for a year of affiliation in at least the four basic services and particularly in obstetrics and pediatrics. The remainder of the course is devoted to some understanding of the behavior, treatment, and nursing of emotionally disturbed persons obtained chiefly through caring for psychotic patients.

Unfortunately this system produces neither a nurse adequately prepared for general bedside nursing, as now practiced in many hospitals, nor one fitted to deal broadly with the most crucial health problem of contemporary society. Anyone acquainted with the public hospital for the mentally ill knows the kinds of patients who fill many of the infirmary beds. Preponderantly they are aged persons, often in advanced stages of cardiac diseases, nephritis, or carcinoma, suffering additionally from senility or other more pronounced mental disturbance. To those educators who believe that initiation into nursing should begin with care of patients who are most nearly well and normal, and that sickness should be viewed as a deviation from the normal, such an environment must seem entirely unsuitable for the training of first-year students. Geriatrics and mental illness are both problems that demand the most thoughtful attention of the nursing as well as the medical profession. But for the student nurse to begin her clinical training in medical and surgical nursing in a setting further confused by the complications of old age and emotional disturbance is an educational experience that we believe should be ended.

The later clinical period, moreover, is necessarily focused upon psychotic patients and their care, rather than upon giving the student a deep understanding of the emotional component of all physical disease. Similarly it fails to prepare her most advantageously to engage in the psychotherapy that has been previously visualized in this report as exceedingly important if disturbances are to be checked in early stages and thus kept from developing into psychoses. At best these schools produce nurses who are skilled in the care of psychotic patients according to the standards of practice in their parent hospitals.

The foregoing statements are not intended to imply that the vast clinical facilities of these institutions should not be used for teaching purposes. Quite the contrary. Many of these 28 hospitals receive students for an affiliation in psychiatric nursing, as do a much larger number of hospitals for the mentally ill, both public and private, that do not conduct schools. There is considerable agreement that public hospitals generally should be used as rapidly as nursing situations suitable for clinical education can be established, but that they should be used for students at an advanced stage of their basic curriculum or for graduate nurses engaged in preparing for specialization in psychiatric nursing. Hence these resources would become available to schools in universities or general hospitals without adequate psychiatric divisions that had arranged for affiliations and had laid the basic foundation for their students to gain the maximum benefit from an experience in psychiatric nursing.

One of the most encouraging developments in nursing education in recent years is the increased emphasis upon requiring of *all* students some three months of clinical experience in psychiatric nursing. Already this has led to the establishment of affiliations with many hospitals where no such arrangements had formerly existed. The progress of this movement is now retarded primarily by the fact that better clinical nursing and better supervision are necessary in some hospitals before schools wish to send students there.

Although nursing education as a whole has many bewildering problems with which to deal, it should attempt to extend every possible assistance to those state hospitals that would be willing to work toward substituting a system of affiliations for present unsatisfactory schools of nursing. In no area of the health services have the nursing and medical professions, as well as the public, so distinct a challenge as in hospitals for the mentally ill. The administrative staff of many state hospitals continuously makes a plea for public interest and help in converting them from primarily custodial institutions into real hospitals where every curative and remedial resource available, including adequate nursing care, is actively utilized.

Except for a negligible number of truly valiant efforts, such as those exerted through the United States Public Health Service, or by the National Committee for Mental Hygiene and the more recent National Mental Health Foundation, the public is largely apathetic. Its interest in a malady that fills approximately half of all hospital beds is far less than in cancer or heart disease. The medical profession is similarly uninterested in state hospitals and the plight of their patients. Endlessly it announces that medical care in the United States is the best in the world. If every physician were required to serve in a hospital for the mentally ill for a time, he might conclude that silence about the level of medical care, comparative or otherwise, would be in better taste.

We recommend that hospitals for the mentally ill still conducting schools of nursing consider means whereby they can relinquish their schools and, as a substitute, make their clinical facilities more widely available for affiliating students. We recommend also that the nursing

136

*profession, both autonomously and in conjunction with the medical pro-
fession and the public at large, attempt to redress the imbalance resulting
from long neglect of mental disease by assisting these and other similar
hospitals to introduce substantial teaching programs for affiliation or
internship and to utilize in-service training for assistant personnel more
extensively and effectively. We recommend particularly that ways be
sought to stimulate interest among the health professions in wider practice
in the field of psychiatric as contrasted with other disease, and in wider
research in its prevention and cure.*

Additional kinds of specialized hospitals that operate schools of
nursing are public tuberculosis sanatoriums and voluntary children's hospitals. There are now only four state-accredited schools
in sanatoriums. In January 1948 their total enrollment was 80.
Many of the same problems that characterize schools in public
hospitals for the mentally ill are found in these schools. *It is our
opinion that their clinical facilities too should be used exclusively for the training of students from other schools that seek affiliations in tuberculosis nursing.*

The three voluntary children's hospitals that operate schools
are well-known institutions. One has maintained a school for
almost sixty years which would certainly be ranked among the
leading hospital schools. Even the youngest school, located in the
Rocky Mountain area, is almost forty years old. These schools
have no such insuperable or numerous problems as besiege
schools in hospitals for the mentally ill. Their principal problem
is that of providing sufficiently varied clinical experience for
their students. Enrollment in one school is now slightly more than
100 students; in each of the other two it barely exceeds 50. All
three receive students from other schools for affiliation in pediatric nursing. It has already been noted that pediatrics is a
service in which many general hospitals are so weak that their
schools must arrange for students to receive experience in this
specialty elsewhere. *The question, therefore, should be raised of whether
the future function of these particular hospitals does not lie entirely in
providing affiliation, rather than in attempting to operate small schools.*

VI

EDUCATION FOR THE PROFESSIONAL NURSE

ALMOST without a dissenting voice those who are conversant with the trend of professional education in the United States agree that preparation of the professional nurse belongs squarely within the institution of higher learning. So convinced are they that they consider this conclusion above argument.

NEED FOR BOTH ACADEMIC AND PROFESSIONAL TRAINING

Two distinct but closely interrelated kinds of preparation that only higher education is broadly equipped to provide are essential for the making of such a nurse. The first is the laying of a foundation that permits continuing growth of many kinds, such as in: positive health and integration of the personality; insight into one's own motivation, the behavior of others, and cultural patterns that condition human behavior; ability to use spoken and written language effectively as a method of communication[1]; skill in analysis of problems, methods of obtaining needed data, and formulation of logical conclusions, principles, or theories; perspective, gained from the historical and anthropological record of human development, of contemporary social institutions and their functions; understanding of and conviction about

[1] A delightful and convincing argument for language as the greatest invention in human history, and for the advantage held by those who can use words effectively over those who are only technicians, no matter how proficient, appeared in an anonymous article in Harper's Magazine, August 1945, pp. 167–174, entitled "Letter to a Seventeen-Year-Old Son." For the very reason that nursing education must cultivate in students far greater skill in the use of words and conceptual thinking than has been undertaken as yet, many schools of nursing would probably like to make excerpts from this article available for faculty and student consideration and discussion.

138

the rights and responsibilities of intelligent citizenship and membership in a profession.

The second kind of preparation is the more specifically technical training for professional practice. But this training must transcend that for the care of the hospitalized sick. It must be preparation for the broad field of community nursing service. Besides the other relatively well-defined components of the course of study, should be included understanding of the effect of nutrition, housing, employment, economic income, class and caste structure, recreational activities, and so forth, upon individual and national health; some knowledge of the principles and functions of social work and of how nurses and social workers can most effectively act as a team; experiments in analyzing the health needs of individuals, families, and communities, and in initiating action to meet these needs; and preparation in the art of teaching health to persons, whether sick or well and whether individually or in groups.[1]

Some readers will conclude from the two preceding paragraphs that an educational pattern is being advocated that is pretentious and on an unnecessarily high level. The worst fears of those who maintain that nurses are being overeducated will seem to be justified. It must therefore be recalled that this is the preparation proposed for that relatively small segment of nurses who should

[1] The writer regrets that the scope of her assignment does not permit description of these and other constituent parts of the two interrelated kinds of preparation. The reader is referred, however, to Nursing by Lulu K. Wolf, of the Vanderbilt University School of Nursing (New York, D. Appleton-Century Co., 1947). The thesis of Professor Wolf's book (Preface, p. v) is that every nurse who assumes the care of a patient "has an obligation to him, his family, and the community in which he lives, to conserve his health and prevent further illness. Not only must the nurse care for the patient during illness and help him get well, but she must care for him in such a way that he will stay well after he gets well." On this thesis she has built an argument for and an analysis of a form of nursing education that encompasses either explicitly or implicitly nearly everything noted above. It is believed that persons interested in this encouraging broader orientation toward the function of nursing will profit from the book. Certain portions might desirably be lengthened and still further deepened in meaning and then presented to the public without those chapters on the techniques of patient care which, however excellent, lead the laity to believe that the book was prepared exclusively for nurses.

be expected to act in truly professional capacities. At the expense
of repeating what was said in an earlier chapter, let us look again
at the functions which only professional nurses are competent to
perform and ask whether anything short of what has been suggested can provide adequate preparation.

These are nurses who will be expected to be fully contributing
team members in complex clinical situations, where both technical skill of a high order and psychological and sociological
orientation are requisite; in the wide field of community nursing
and community health services where prevention of disease and
therapy, but more particularly the maintenance of health, are
ever-widening goals; in the supervision of the activities of many
kinds of assistant and graduate personnel; in planning and administering nursing programs, often within agencies and institutions of great size and complicated organizational structure. Included also are those nurses who must assume responsibility for
formulating educational programs; instructing students of nursing, graduate nurses, practical nurses, and other assistant
personnel in the content and methodology of nursing, and in
what the student and graduate nurse should teach patients individually and in groups and how this can best be done; carrying
on desperately needed research, writing, publication, and consultation related to the improvement and extension of nursing
care; planning for the continued growth and development of the
nursing profession; and administering those plans in close cooperation with other health services and with the needs of society
always in mind.

INTEGRATION OF ACADEMIC AND PROFESSIONAL CURRICULA

We conclude that education for such nurses cannot be adequate unless it includes generous portions of both kinds of preparation outlined. It is essential to build a base that will foster a
developmental process extending throughout life. To the extent

that these two kinds of preparation are interwoven, student motivation and understanding are likely to be enhanced and the time necessary for establishing the foundation reduced.

Attempts at such integration have not largely characterized most professional education in the United States. Instead, the professional school, whether in law, medicine, social work, or library work, has customarily made a specified length of time spent in the undergraduate college (two, three, or four years as the case may be) a prerequisite for admission. It has proceeded on the assumption that the function of the liberal arts college is to provide the first kind of preparation, and that it can therefore concentrate its attention upon technical training.

This pattern was followed until recently by most university schools of nursing which established basic curricula. Two years of college, with certain required courses in English, the physiological, biological, and sometimes social sciences, constituted the general requirement for admission, although two schools insisted for a time on the bachelor's degree and one continues to do so. Thus the degree-conferring school of nursing was supposedly free to devote itself exclusively to the professional curriculum which most frequently was three calendar years in length, like that of the hospital school.

Of late, professional schools of several kinds have begun to question the desirability of this sharp separation between liberal arts and professional education. They recognize that some undergraduate colleges give excellent preparation in the obtaining, interpreting, and integrating of knowledge, and in helping students to advance to an adult level of experience and responsibility. On such a beginning they can construct their professional training advantageously. But far more often they discover, even when they require academic preparation in certain designated fields, that students come to them with such diverse and strange assortments of knowledge of a purely descriptive and unrelated kind, and with almost no preparation in the methodology of

141

finding and using data, that little is contributed to their professional training. As a consequence they must either attempt, as many of them are now doing to some degree, to build into the curriculum relevant portions of general education, or they must continue instruction which is robbed of the depth and significance essential for the preparation of professional, as contrasted with vocational, persons. Hence they conclude that the dichotomy in higher education is wasteful and expensive, and often tends to retard rather than promote development toward adulthood.

This characteristic pattern of separation of general and professional education has not been followed in the field of engineering. Students have always been received into schools of engineering directly from secondary schools. Almost without exception the basic curriculum has been four academic years in length, and it has led to a bachelor's degree in one of several types of engineering of which the most common are civil, mechanical, electrical, and chemical. The course of study has invariably been "stiff" for the majority of students. Often their summers have been spent gaining experience in industry.

Engineering schools have long been recognized as institutions with carefully defined and conscientiously taught curricula, capable of producing graduates with a high degree of technical proficiency. Elective courses have been relatively few. Choice permitted the student has been primarily that of selecting the particular field of engineering in which he wished to concentrate during his last two years. The shortcoming of these schools has lain in their failure to include enough related general education to give their graduates parity with lawyers, economists, or bankers, for example, in the use of language as a tool for communication, to acquaint them sufficiently with the nature and purposes of society within which they must live and work, and to help them adequately with interpersonal relationships.

During the past quarter of this century concerted effort has been undertaken in many schools to lessen these deficiencies. The very fact that engineers have entered managerial positions whether in engineering enterprises or in industry in progressively larger numbers, has indirectly encouraged these schools to enlarge their offerings in general education. Some have lengthened their curricula from four to five years. Others have introduced the perhaps more valuable experiment of including needed general courses within the four-year period. As a result the curriculum would be so overcrowded it could not bear the strain if continuing attention were not focused on keeping the technical courses pared to the barest fundamentals and most basic problems. Initial attempts have also been made to improve teaching methods to such an extent that each course (English, history, or psychology, as well as technical courses) will not only be useful to learning in subsequent courses, but will carry forward prior learning by drawing upon what was previously taught.[1]

INTEGRATION AS A PATTERN FOR FUTURE NURSING EDUCATION

The kind of preparation for the professional nurse that nurse educators have now come to advocate is strikingly like that provided by schools of engineering. Students are to be admitted directly from high school to a basic curriculum that is the product of attempts to integrate general and technical training. The length of the course usually recommended is approximately four calendar, not academic, years including vacations of one month annually. The recognition to be granted is generally the degree of Bachelor of Science in Nursing.

[1] Nurse educators concerned with integration of the curriculum and teaching methods would probably like to make available for study a paper entitled "Professional Education in a Free Society," read on February 14, 1946 by Elliott Dunlap Smith, provost and professor of social relations at the Carnegie Institute of Technology, Pittsburgh. It is primarily a discussion of the relative functions of general and of technical courses within an integrated curriculum, and of how the several courses in the two types of training may be used to advance each other. Dr. Smith's professional preparation was not in engineering, but in law and psychology.

A number of schools already exist that have introduced the integrated program or are moving toward its introduction. A few are new schools established since nursing education made this reorientation in its philosophy; others are schools that have revised or are revising their structure and curricula. The writer visited several such schools in the United States and one in Canada. At present the picture is often badly confused by situations like the following. Considerable numbers of students are admitted after having had two years of college elsewhere. Diploma courses are still found although decreasingly in some of these schools, and degree students and diploma students are given clinical experience, at least, together. Educational efforts are seriously dissipated by having to provide "advanced programs" for graduate nurses, who need to make up deficiencies in general and technical training. Under these circumstances it is not surprising that coordination between the two parts of the curriculum has not reached a more advanced stage of development than is sometimes found.

These schools are in no such favorable position as are engineering schools that receive large financial support from the university, that can depend upon having about all the carefully selected students they wish to enroll, and that are generally free to give their exclusive attention to building basic curricula for such students. Many of the difficulties of these nursing schools will be solved, however, as fast as qualified students are attracted in sufficient numbers, and a budget comparable to that of other professional schools is provided for them. They will then be left with the hardest task still before them: that of achieving true integration of subject matter and of teaching methods. That task will require much time, patience, and the cooperative efforts of nurse and other university instructors. But to any extent that integration is attained, improvement over the fragmentation of knowledge that characterizes American education will be demonstrated.

144

Experiments in the Integrated Curriculum

Because the integrated basic curriculum of four calendar years represents the pattern that is now being forged for the future, on the basis of which subsequent planning for the preparation of professional nurses should probably move forward, a brief description will be given of two experiments. They will provide the lay reader with at least a cursory picture of the nature of this kind of curriculum.

The first experiment was begun nearly twenty-five years ago. Although it was established within a woman's college rather than a university, the college offers not only the customary liberal arts program but seven specialized curricula, all of which lead to a bachelor's degree. The curriculum is four calendar years in length. The first and fourth academic years are spent on the college campus, the remainder of the time in hospitals and nursing agencies. During the first academic year the following courses are required: English, anatomy and physiology, microbiology, chemistry, general and educational psychology, foods and nutrition, and more briefly child study and physical education.

Subsequently the students are introduced, for a sixteen week summer session, to the main hospital laboratory. There they receive instruction and supervised practice in elementary nursing and in the care of convalescent patients. One comprehensive course, introduction to nursing, and small courses in drugs and solutions, pharmacology and therapeutics, and introduction to medical and surgical nursing are required. At the end of this summer session any students who lack aptitude for or interest in nursing may withdraw and return to the college to enter other fields of study.

The second year is devoted to instruction and supervised practice both in the in-patient and outpatient departments of the main hospital, with its rich teaching facilities in medicine, surgery, and pediatrics. In addition to courses related to nursing in these three fields, formal instruction is given in professional

145

adjustments, diet therapy, and social and health aspects of nursing.

Three other hospitals provide the laboratories to which third-year students are assigned for periods ranging from two to four months in neuropsychiatric, tuberculosis, and obstetrical nursing. The main hospital also provides two additional months of medical and surgical nursing.

For the academic portion of the fourth year the students again return to the college campus. The two-semester senior conference permits opportunity for a survey of the field of nursing, particularly of contemporary trends. Two semesters of introductory sociology, history, and English are required. Except for history of nursing and physical education, the remainder of the course of study is elective.

The program is concluded with a senior nursing period of sixteen weeks. Half of that time must be devoted to urban family health service in a visiting nurse association. For the remaining two months the student may elect further training in any one of the more customary hospital services, including psychiatry, obstetrics, and tuberculosis, or in urban or rural family health service. If she prefers, she may assist a selected head nurse in unit management and teaching how to give planned care to patients. She will be expected to participate in many small group conferences concerned with understanding of the patient's behavior and meeting his needs.

The second experiment is that of a school which is an integral part of one of Canada's leading universities. In 1942 a degree course of four years was introduced. It was lengthened in 1946 to five years, thus permitting inclusion of more study of the humanities, better integration of the professional and academic subjects throughout the curriculum, smoother and sounder clinical practice, more time for growth in intellectual and emotional comprehension, and longer vacations than those provided by other schools of nursing.

The first year is devoted to English, history, psychology, chemistry, biology, and an unbroken course in introduction to nursing. This course begins with class work in the first term, includes practice in skills in the second, and develops into two months of daily hospital practice at the end. In the second year English, history, and nursing are continued. The nursing course centers attention on the theory and practice of medical and surgical nursing and public health nursing. Three new subjects are added: philosophy, physiology, and an introductory course in preventive medicine that includes laboratory work in bacteriology.

The third year consists to a considerable degree of preparation in the customary clinical subjects and in the theory and field practice of public health nursing. English, philosophy, and the sciences, nevertheless, are scheduled. In the fourth year theory and practice in public health nursing and in clinical subjects are continued; nutrition, social casework, and education are also required. The fifth year, as designed at present, will include nursing (probably ward management), preventive medicine, sociology, education, and psychology.

Annotations on this course of study prepared by the director of the school and published in the annual bulletin emphasize the nature and extent of the integration attempted within the curriculum. Although clinical experience in medical and surgical nursing is provided at particular periods, almost every other hospital service—whether pediatrics, obstetrics, tuberculosis, or psychiatry—affords continued practice in medical or in surgical nursing or in both. Mental hygiene, nutrition, and public health or preventive medicine are subjects to which specific courses are devoted. They are also associated "at all times," writes the director, with the teaching of nursing and with nursing practice. Similarly sociology and methods of social work are presented in individual courses, but their principles are constantly drawn on in the theory and practice of nursing and in preventive medicine.

147

A particular attempt is being made to define the field where "social work and medicine meet," and to prepare students for practice in that area.[1] Special attention is given through courses in education and by less formal means to help the student begin a critical appreciation of sound principles of general and professional education. Preparation for teaching is offered at intervals during several years.

Integration is also fostered by the method of instruction utilized. Every member of the faculty who teaches nursing to undergraduate students must be prepared to teach in both classroom and ward. Furthermore, she must be prepared to teach the preventive and curative aspects of every phase of nursing, the mental as well as the physical aspects of patient care, and the nutritional and dietetic aspects.

This university school maintains affiliations with some eight general and specialized hospitals and with a considerable list of public health and social agencies. As in the instance of the first school described, one large hospital serves as the laboratory for a prolonged period of experience in several nursing services. Thereafter, the rich clinical facilities of specialized hospitals and of several agencies are utilized.

Inherent Advantages

Many advantages of integration have been indicated in the foregoing pages. Attention must be called specifically to two that merit particular interest. The first is that integration provides a method for putting an end to the preclinical period which char-

[1] Several college and university schools of nursing in the United States require one course in social work, primarily because of the help it will supposedly give the nurse in her practice and in cooperative undertakings with social workers. At present there is some discussion, still only in an exploratory phase, of the desirability of preparing a person who could combine public health nursing and common social work skills sufficiently to act both as a nurse and a social worker. Such a person is to be found in practice in many countries. Particularly in the rural areas of the United States and Canada, which suffer from a dearth of professional personnel of all kinds and where any considerable number of social workers is not likely to be available in the near future, it is thought that this combined function might serve an exceedingly useful purpose.

acterizes all hospital schools and also most collegiate schools that accept students with two years of liberal arts. How truly constructive educational experience can be given within the confines of that brief preclinical period which is a vestigial survival of the old system of probation is a problem that no school, despite earnest effort and radical improvement, has solved satisfactorily.

The establishment of a propitious substitute, however, has not been easy or entirely successful. Anyone acquainted with higher education knows only too well the inadequacies of subject matter and the lack of interest in cultivating new areas that often exist among university professors. Hence it would be naive to assume that fruitful cooperative relations between the faculty of nursing and those of the larger parent body can always be established with facility. Academic courses required of nursing students in integrated curricula still fall far short in many places of providing the help needed. Nevertheless a plan has been devised that permits distinct hope of achieving a larger competence than has been possible within the framework of the preclinical period.

The second advantage to be emphasized is that integration provides a challenge to experimentation. Its very newness and its creative possibilities are strong stimulants, to a profession weary from the heavy weight of traditionalism, to fashion a form of educational preparation more nearly in conformity with contemporary requirements, and contemporary principles of education and curriculum construction.

One of the most promising aspects of nursing education that the writer encountered in several places in her trip around the country was the enthusiasm, initiative, and originality with which nurse educators of first-rate ability were striving to design, restudy, or refashion the curriculum as a whole, and every course in it, within a conceptual pattern of total needs. The sharpness of the contrast between this truly professional approach to education and that of harassed directors and their assistants, who

149

conceived of a curriculum largely as something more to be administered, rather than something to be created, can scarcely be visualized by those who have not visited schools of nursing extensively.

Wherever this creativeness was found, it recalled those two questions that have so often been raised about nursing. Can nursing develop a specific content of its own, thus establishing a larger claim to professionalism? Will nurse educators ever engage in any considerable amount of research and writing which for some universities is the hallmark of the right to be included within the fraternity of higher education? The writer was convinced that the day would not be far distant, if what is now occurring in a few centers were extended to many more, when both these questions could be answered squarely in the affirmative.

Because this broad generalization appears within a discussion of the integrated curriculum, no one should conclude that creativeness was found only within schools that have introduced that type of education. Forward-looking and imaginative undertakings in improving the nature and content of the curriculum were evident in several university schools that admit students only for the professional curriculum in nursing, and in hospital schools of the kind designated as belonging within the university. For the very reason, however, that the integrated curriculum permits coordination of both kinds of preparation and facilitates logical enrichment of the entire course of study, it probably provides the largest encouragement to and reward for experimentation.

We recommend that as new basic curricula are established within institutions of higher learning or as existing curricula are fundamentally altered, careful consideration be given to the possible advantages of utilizing the pattern of organizational structure laid down by engineering schools and already introduced in nursing education, rather than the pattern that has characterized most of professional education. In order that these integrated basic curricula may have the maximum opportunity for growth and development and for proving themselves, *we recommend, further, that competing diploma courses be completely eliminated, and that advanced programs for graduate nurses* (who need very different preparation from that required by basic students and for whom considerable provision already exists) *be continued only if they do not detract from the time, attention, and financial resources that should be devoted to building basic curricula.*[1]

Requirements for Establishing Sound Professional Schools of Nursing

Thus far it has been noted that considerable amounts of academic, as well as technical education, must be provided as a basis for contemporary professional practice. The suggestion has been made that the integrated curriculum probably offers the most efficient means to achieve this end. But there are several other important considerations that must be kept clearly in view if sound professional education is to result.

Organizational Structure

Whether the curriculum be of the integrated or the purely professional type, it is essential that the organizational structure of the school be clear cut and designed to facilitate the development of the program. At present a confusing variety of forms of organization exists, some of which are of doubtful validity. They reflect the various efforts made to establish nursing education within the university or college. Only the two most common forms need concern us: completely independent administrative units on a parity with other professional schools in the institution of higher learning; separate departments or schools generally within the college of liberal arts but sometimes within a medical college or other division.

[1] Reference will be made later to provision for true graduate work and professional education on the higher levels.

The writer was told by two directors that the fact that their schools were under the jurisdiction of colleges of liberal arts had been a source of strength and help in the early days of these particular schools and of nursing education within institutions of higher learning. In each instance the dean of the college provided sympathetic understanding and wise counsel to the school, and lent his prestige and procedural knowledge in making representation of its interests before the president of the university. After nearly twenty years within the college, one of these schools has recently been reorganized as a completely independent unit. Its dean occupies a chair beside the deans of medicine, dentistry, and pharmacy in the councils of the Board of Health Sciences where policies are formulated for the four schools, and she has direct access to the office of the president, exactly like all other deans in the university.

Since nursing education was first established in universities and colleges, much experience has been gained in regard to its function and place there. The content of the curriculum and teaching methods have been greatly expanded and improved. Although still far too small, the number of nurse educators prepared to grapple with problems of administration is much larger than formerly. Hence less justification can today be found for other than the completely independent form of organizational structure.

Such autonomy, moreover, is conducive—if not now almost necessary—to the further promotion of nursing education. The school must be prepared to meet competitive situations within the university generally, but more particularly in its relations with the medical school and the hospitals from which clinical facilities are obtained. For this reason it is important that the school be accorded the same recognition as other professional schools, and that the director be given the status of dean and a seat at the conference table on the highest executive level.

Some universities have raised the question of whether they could rightfully make schools of nursing of correlative importance with other professional schools, when it is almost impossible to find nurses who hold the doctorate to fill even the directorship. This question has been asked before when other new professions have sought to gain access to the institution of higher learning. Yet the doctorate has rarely been used as a criterion for the selection either of dean or faculty in such well-established professions as engineering and law. There are probably many schools of engineering where no one yet holds a degree higher than the master's. Few of the most outstanding professors of law have an earned doctorate, and not more than a half dozen law schools award such a degree. In both of these professions experience gained through practice has consistently been considered more important than graduate work.

If in the near future universities should make the doctorate a prerequisite for the deanship or for full professorial rank, nursing education might be seriously retarded. If, on the other hand, universities select the best persons available and then grant full support and recognition to their schools of nursing, it is believed that nursing education will move ahead with such rapidity that a generation hence even persons with the doctorate will be available, should the degree still seem of major importance.

We recommend that schools created in the future within institutions of higher learning be made autonomous units vested with the same status as the other professional schools, and that schools already in existence that are not fully independent be helped to become so.

Facilities

The few inadequately equipped classrooms and laboratories housed within a nurses' residence, which the visitor to hospital schools of nursing so often finds, are a symbol of the kind of provision that has generally characterized nursing education in the United States. The school of nursing is reminiscent of the outpatient service, to which reference has already been made. Both have suffered gravely from lack of even a location that would offer dignity, physical comfort, and cheerfulness.

Hospitals and nurses' residences constructed in recent years have generally shown decided improvement in the facilities and equipment provided the nursing school. Nevertheless education has continued to be centered in the nurses' residence, with the hospital used as a practice laboratory. So persistent has been this pattern that it has even been carried over into some universities that had never considered putting the home economics "practice house," for example, within a dormitory.

In general, however, the university has tended to provide better physical facilities than have most hospital schools. Well-established educational institutions usually consider it an obligation to maintain good standards relating to physical plant and to equipment, as well as to libraries and other cultural resources that serve all faculties and students. Such institutions are usually unwilling to open new professional schools unless they can guarantee the continuance of those standards.

Largely as the result of historical developments and pressures to which they have been subjected, however, universities have almost unconsciously evolved patterns of larger aid to, and concern for, some parts of their institutions than others. Agriculture, engineering, the physical sciences, and medicine have been especially favored recipients. Nursing, which is new to the campus and speaks in a voice that is still weak, is often regarded as a "poor relation" who finds herself on the periphery of activities, both physically and psychologically. Because the professional nurse is of such preeminent importance to society, it would appear unquestionable that the university should move steadily toward providing facilities for her education more nearly on a level with those provided the medical student. Administrators of nursing education, moreover, should learn to make their requests for university consideration more forceful; else they will not be heard among the voices of the other deans.

But university facilities other than those supplied directly to the school of nursing need to be utilized to the fullest degree possible. Because nursing has suffered greatly in the past from isolation within hospital walls, it is essential that the collegiate school be made an integral part of the university environment. One of the advantages of having the school in the university, rather than in a hospital able to give excellent instruction, is the opportunity provided for contact with persons whose primary focus of attention is education. Students of nursing who are subsequently to act in capacities where the intellectual component is large, must be given a chance, like the members of every other profession, to learn how to engage in that intellectual process. The best means available is through participation with teachers and students from many fields who are attempting to be articulate about ideas, and through sharing in the resources provided by the university to aid in intellectual growth and development.

Few professional schools take full advantage of what the university affords in lectures, libraries, exhibitions, concerts, or discussion groups. Yet where intra-university contacts have been larger and more fertile, a heartening vitality and expanded frame of intellectual reference have been seen. Consequently while nursing education in the university is still young enough for new patterns to be more easily established, and the integrated curriculum offers exceptionally rich opportunity for fostering contacts among various departments, especial effort should be given to bring the school within the orbit of university thought and activities.

Like the medical school, the nursing school must have not only classroom, laboratory, and cultural facilities, but also resources for the various kinds of clinical experience necessary for the preparation of professional personnel. These resources the university may or may not provide directly. Fortunate indeed is the school that exists within a university which operates a large teaching hospital for medical students with well-diversified clinical services, and which has for teaching purposes the use of specialized hospitals and agencies. Under such circumstances the obtaining of good clinical facilities is relatively easy.

Present standards of nursing education applicable to college students demand that resources be available for teaching in the four basic services, and in communicable disease, psychiatric, and public health nursing. As has been noted experience is also being increasingly sought in nursery schools or child development centers where the student may study normal growth and development. In some places field experience in both rural and urban public health nursing is being fostered, and affiliations with community and rural hospitals are being encouraged. These last types of student experience are likely to undergo large development in future years.

To the extent that the university itself does not provide requisite clinical facilities, relations must be established with hospitals and agencies which should be formalized through signed contracts. A distinct advantage of the university school is its potentially greater freedom than the hospital school enjoys to select those clinical facilities needed. That university schools have not always used this opportunity to best advantage is undoubtedly true. Evidence implicit in the earlier reports of the two integrated curricula or in other reports that could be cited demonstrate, however, the success achieved by some schools in obtaining clinical resources that are rich and well diversified, and that supply students with experience within different environmental situations and with health nursing as well as sick nursing.

In this connection the writer wishes to digress for a moment to pay tribute to the deans of two university schools she has visited, who have seen an opportunity to obtain ample clinical experience for their students, and simultaneously to begin improvement of nursing services in hospitals under consideration. These institutions were public general hospitals or state hospitals for the mentally ill. Their clinical resources were almost limitless, but the nursing care provided was on an exceedingly unsatisfactory level. They were eager to be used for teaching purposes, for thus considerable influence would be exerted, it was thought, over their nursing practices generally. The problem lay in their ability to create even a few nursing units within the vast services well enough staffed and equipped so that they could be used for clinical instruction. At the time of the visits, such attempts were being undertaken with the consultative help of the two university schools. In both instances the head of the school had her eyes directed not only to the needs of nursing students, but to that other important professional task of improvement of nursing service through demonstration of what constitutes good care and supervision of the patient.

This is not the appropriate place to engage in a detailed discussion of procedural questions relating to contractual arrangements between the university school of nursing and hospitals and agencies utilized for clinical teaching. One general principle, however, must be kept clearly in mind. The university school should enter into relations with other institutions exclusively to obtain necessary clinical laboratories, not to help provide nursing service for patients. Regrettably, some university schools find themselves in the same situation as most hospital schools, where students are expected to supply nursing care at the expense of the educational process.

Two major reasons are responsible for this difficulty. First, the average hospital, reared in the tradition of depending upon nursing students for much of the care of patients, does not yet exhibit the same attitude toward the school of nursing as toward the medical school. It expects little service from medical students. Yet it welcomes the opportunity to be a teaching hospital for a medical school, for it knows that thereby its prestige will be enhanced and its standards of medical practice will be maintained and probably raised. That the university should help the hospital to view the school of nursing in a similar fashion appears

157

to be part of the responsibility to be assumed by any institution of higher learning which undertakes the professional education of nurses.

The second reason is that the financial resources of many university schools and their students are so small that additional sources of revenue must be found. Hence a school sometimes helps to maintain itself through contracting for reimbursement for nursing service provided by students. In almost all instances students earn their board and room by supplying nursing care. Under such circumstances the demands of service are likely to be placed before the demands of education.

During recent months one nationally known school has succeeded, it believes, in putting its financial arrangements with the university hospital on a sounder basis. Students are no longer responsible to the hospital, but only to the school, during the time allotted to education. Hence the hospital can make no demand for service exceeding what the clinical instructors believe essential for educational purposes. In turn students are required to pay for their own maintenance. Because most of them need to earn money to cover living expenses, the school has arranged for them to work as employes of the hospital for one four-hour evening each week and also for eight hours on Saturday or Sunday, when hospitals generally experience their worst difficulty in obtaining adequate nursing care. As compensation the hospital pays them an hourly sum intermediate between that paid the trained practical and the graduate nurse. This plan for separating service and education more distinctly and formally may prove of considerable usefulness to other universities struggling with a similar problem.

However, it is doubtful whether the fundamental question of contractual arrangements between university and hospital or agency can be settled with any large degree of permanent satisfaction until much more financial support is made available to nursing education.

We recommend that the university which now operates or subsequently establishes a school of nursing make substantial effort to provide it with physical accommodations and equipment comparable to that provided other professional schools on the campus requiring laboratory and practice facilities, and that plans be drawn to bring it as completely as possible within the intellectual and cultural orbit of the parent institution.

Second, we recommend that the university seek the best available clinical facilities in whatever number is deemed desirable for the promotion of sound professional education; that relations established between the university and hospitals and agencies be formalized through written contracts which detail the respective privileges and obligations of the two contracting parties, including as incisive a statement as can be negotiated concerning the use of the student's time exclusively for purposes of education.

Faculty

Sound basic principles concerning the faculty of schools that are parts of institutions of higher learning have been formulated by the Association of Collegiate Schools of Nursing. These principles, which include reference to appointment, status, qualifications, and the teaching and administrative load, appear in the following paragraphs:

There shall be a well-organized, competent faculty, adequate in number to carry out effectively the educational program offered.

The faculty shall have academic status in accord with the policy governing faculty organization in that college or university of which the school is a part.

The qualifications of members of the faculty and regular teaching staff shall be baccalaureate or higher degree from an accredited college and a sound basic professional preparation, supplemented by specialized professional preparation and experience which qualify them in subjects that they teach.

The teaching load of each member of the faculty or teaching staff who carries no administrative duties shall be in accord with the policy of the college or university. The teaching load should be reduced in the case of those who carry administrative responsibilities.

Little needs to be added to this official statement except to say that in interpreting these principles many schools that are members of the Association have already begun to emphasize the master's degree rather than the baccalaureate as a prerequisite for appointment to any faculty position above the level of instructor. The trend is obviously toward making the master's degree a minimum qualification in schools that are expected to maintain standards generally comparable to those of other schools on the campus.

The phenomenal progress achieved in the past two decades in equipping nurses with a broader academic and professional background for teaching is profoundly encouraging. How enough nurses can be prepared to staff existent and prospective schools, however, is still one of the critical problems faced by nursing education. The problem is made more acute by the fact that several other nursing specialties besides teaching compete for the services of those persons who have had advanced preparation.

Of the schools visited in the late summer of 1947, scarcely one had been able to complete its teaching roster for the September term. Directors were often urgently attempting to learn by telegram of persons whom they might interest in available positions. In spite of all efforts the result was the same as in preceding years: many positions went unfilled or were filled by nurses who failed to have the qualifications desired.

Reference has already been made to the reason for this dearth of nurses with as much as a bachelor's degree: the shortsightedness of a system of hospital training that has shown little interest in planning for the leadership and future growth and development of the profession. In 1947 only six out of every 100 students entering schools of nursing were enrolled in a program leading to a degree. The other 94 were enrolled in a diploma program, and only one of them had completed four years of college. The picture differed appreciably from state to state. In the jurisdiction with the most favorable record probably about one in every five

160

students was registered in a degree-conferring school; in 15 jurisdictions not one such school existed.

Until such time as the number of students completing basic degree programs is vastly increased, attention must obviously be placed upon helping graduate nurses to obtain the baccalaureate. Simultaneously preparation on higher levels must be forwarded as rapidly as possible. In 1945 there were 46 universities and colleges that offered "advanced programs" leading to a degree for students who were already R.N.s. Of these 31 specialized in preparation only for the baccalaureate; 15 offered additional preparation for the master's degree. The total number is probably larger now.

Because statistics have never been collected for the number of graduate nurses registered in advanced programs, figures are not available either for total enrollments or for distribution according to the specific degree sought. Two universities, however, attract a large proportion of the graduate nurses pursuing advanced work. In one of them a recent count showed almost 1,000 students enrolled on a full-time or part-time basis; 532 were known to be registered for the baccalaureate degree, 237 for the master's degree, and 9 for the doctorate. Others were unclassified. Between October 1946 and October 1947, this university had conferred the B.S. on 122 nurses, M.A. on 97, M.S. on one, and Ph.D. on one. The second university had a total registration of 1,255, of whom 1,028 were classified as undergraduate students, 153 were working for the master's degree, and 13 for the doctorate. The remainder were not registered for a degree.

Considerable criticism exists of advanced programs as they are operated. Some persons maintain that preparation is frequently offered in various fields of clinical teaching and supervision, for example, that cannot be justified on the basis of the clinical facilities, faculty, and funds available. Others complain that too large a proportion of these programs consists of didactic courses in methods of teaching, that are insufficiently dynamic and broad in scope and that are required at the expense of courses dealing with content. Still others insist that these curricula fail, for other than financial reasons, to attract many of the most promising students. Finally, there is the widespread criticism that much of the work offered is "advanced" in name only. It must be recalled, however, that basic training is frequently so inadequate that programs for the graduate nurse must first seek to eliminate deficiencies in the earlier preparation.

The degree of validity of these criticisms is not known, since a comprehensive study of advanced curricula has not been undertaken. Such a study is greatly needed. Perhaps it is only second in importance to examination of schools offering the basic curriculum. Information of the kind that can be collected by distribution of questionnaires would be useful; field examination, university by university, would yield larger results.

But something far more fundamental is needed. It is reformulation of philosophy concerning preparation for teaching and the other nursing specialties, and development of a plan on a nationwide basis for desirable location of units of instruction, including definition of the kinds of instruction that might most profitably be offered in the individual units. This kind of study would probably reveal that existent programs are not always well distributed for serving the interests of nurses in the several parts of the country, and that they are not always operated by those universities with the richest available resources. Thus the present trend for advanced programs to increase in number without sufficient consideration of more than local needs and interests might be checked.

Through such a study universities might be encouraged to cultivate those particular courses for which they were best fitted without feeling obliged to continue to offer preparation for several kinds of specialization. Almost certainly this exploration would point to the desirability of setting aside a few centers devoted exclusively to the development of truly graduate work.

There faculties would be freed from dissipation of time and energy concomitant to helping graduate nurses prepare for the bachelor's degree. Instead they would be expected to concern themselves through experimental teaching, research, and writing with the further development of content and method for all nursing education, and with producing teachers more fully prepared to staff university schools.

We recommend that standards such as those formulated by the Association of Collegiate Schools of Nursing govern the appointment, status, qualifications, and teaching and administrative load of faculty in professional schools of nursing.

Since the very future of these professional schools is dependent upon the rapid numerical increase and improved qualifications of nursing faculty, *we also recommend that early effort be made to examine comprehensively the present system of advanced preparation, and to plan for such reorganization as might attract more women of ability and provide more substantial preparation for leadership in nursing education and the other nursing specialties.*

Financial Structure

Under the title, "Financial Support and Budget," the Association of Collegiate Schools of Nursing wrote two short paragraphs into its statement of principles:

There shall be a definitely assigned budget sufficient in amount to maintain the school on a level commensurate with that of other professional schools in the college or university. A fair proportion of the school's income shall be derived from some stable source other than student fees.

The head of the school shall be responsible for the preparation and the expenditure of the budget in accord with the policy of the college or university.

These basic principles, which would scarcely be questioned by educators, give little clue to how totally inadequate has been the financial support of nursing education thus far provided. Whether truly professional preparation for nursing can move ahead quickly and successfully depends primarily upon its being able to obtain enough funds and faculty personnel to permit sound growth and substantial expansion. Of the two dilemmas, that of finances is perhaps the more critical. Many nurse educators are of the opinion that if funds were more nearly ample for strengthening advanced curricula, and if scholarships and fellowships were more numerous, the problem of preparation of faculty would lend itself to solution. Grants for further study made available by the federal government through the United States Cadet Nurse Corps, the Federal Security Agency, and the "G. I. Bill of Rights" have brought gratifying numbers into the universities and colleges.

Through an unfortunate historical accident the public has as yet made little provision for the support of nursing education. This is in sharp contrast to the financing of the preparation of teachers for elementary and secondary schools. Education for every child has consistently been viewed as the country's foremost instrumentality for advancing the goals of our national life. So firmly has this belief been held that public and also private funds have been poured not only into a system of schools that seeks to reach into every community, but into large numbers of colleges designed specifically for the training of teachers, and departments of education in public and private universities. The principle of financial support of teacher training is an integral part of the mores of the United States.

Today the nurse probably ranks close to the teacher as a social necessity. If she is not needed so continuously to serve the interests of childhood and adolescence, she is needed at times during the life span of every person. Her role as an indispensable member of the health services engaged in therapy, the prevention of disease, and the protection of health is continuously growing in size and importance.

164

Because of the apprenticeship system of training, however, that has characterized nursing education, the public has assumed little responsibility for, or even given much thought to, the proper financing of the preparation of nurses. In the days when the student nurse was more of an apprentice than she is now, the hospital charged her no tuition or fees. Instead, it paid her a small monthly allowance and provided her a living. Thus she "worked out" whatever she received in education, maintenance, and spending money. She may also have contributed to the budgets of many hospitals.

During recent years when better hospital schools have been attempting to convert the student nurse into a person who more nearly resembles a nursing student, the granting of allowances has declined sharply and the practice of charging at least a small tuition has been introduced widely. Consequently the way in which the student pays for her education has changed to some extent. It is believed, however, that in the average hospital school, the student herself is still responsible for almost the entire cost of her education. The United States Public Health Service found, it will be recalled,[1] in the 20 supposedly representative schools investigated that 88 per cent of the income came from student services, 11 per cent from student fees, and 1 per cent from gifts and miscellaneous sources. When income from student services and fees, and from gifts and endowments do not cover the entire cost of operating the school, hospital funds are also used. These funds come from patient fees, endowments and gifts to the hospital, and in the case of public hospitals, from taxes.

By the time nursing education sought admission to institutions of higher learning, conditions were not propitious for universities and colleges to assume large financial responsibilities. Most of them had already accumulated heavy commitments for continuing programs; many were subjected to extreme pressure for enlargement rather than curtailment of these programs. What was

[1] See p. 48.

more important, however, was the fact that the concept of support of nursing education by institutions of higher learning was not in the mores of America. Like society at large, the university had had little orientation in its thinking toward possible responsibility for the preparation of professional nurses. Under the circumstances the very existence of basic or advanced curricula within a considerable number of universities and colleges is greatly to the credit of the boards and administrators of those institutions, the nursing profession, and a few informed, sincerely concerned lay persons and corporate bodies.

The financial foundation is nevertheless so weak almost everywhere that unless it is greatly strengthened, the professional sector of nursing will be seriously handicapped in making a more substantial contribution to the public welfare. Figures for several of the supposedly best financed university schools, some under private and some under public auspices, were supplied upon request for the preparation of this report. Space is not available for reproducing any considerable part of the data received. Hence statistics will be given for only one school which, because of even small endowment funds, probably ranks relatively high in its financial stability. Several schools reported appreciably larger total income, but many of them also reported larger enrollments. In some, expenditure per student appeared to be actually less; in only a few instances was it conspicuously more, and in none was it double the amount. From the following figures one can gain an impression of how small must be the budgets of schools that are in no such fortunate position as those that submitted data.

For the year ending June 30, 1947 total income in the school under consideration was $88,400, of which $38,650 came from endowment and $49,750 from tuition. The expenditures were $91,950. The student enrollment was 224, of whom 106 were matriculated in the basic curriculum and 118 in the curriculum for graduate nurses. Although it was not possible to separate costs for the two curricula satisfactorily, the approximate expenditure per student in the basic curriculum for the year was $470.

The comparison between these figures and those for the medical school of the same university is interesting. The latter, with a student body of 194, had an income of $576,940 and expenditures of $653,600. Hence it spent close to $3,370 on the education of each medical student.[1] Differences in the proportions of expense borne by the two types of students are sharp. The tuition paid by the nursing student during the fiscal year 1946–1947 was only $200. That paid by the medical student during the academic year was $500. The former amount, however, constituted 42.5 per cent of the cost of her education; the latter amount constituted less than 15 per cent of what was spent on the average medical student. For the fiscal year 1948–1949 the tuition of nursing students will be raised to $360; that of medical students only to $600.

The question of paramount importance for the future is how funds are to be obtained whereby institutions of higher learning may catch up on what should have been done much earlier in supporting the preparation of professional nurses. Certainly in this rich country with its tradition of private generosity to the public good, many individuals could and would contribute to nursing education, as they have contributed for example to medical education, if they understood that not only nursing but the health services generally are being retarded by lack of funds for basic professional training. A quarter of a century ago one foundation and one interested woman created small endowment funds for three university nursing schools in the United States. This act has exerted influence disproportionate to the sums given in emphasizing the place of nursing within higher education. The

[1] Figures collected for 1947–1948 by the Council on Medical Education and Hospitals indicate that in 77 schools, 7 of which maintained only the first two years of the medical course, the expenditure per medical student, excluding research funds from outside sources, was as follows: 12 schools spent between $600 and $1,000; 51 spent between $1,000 and $2,500; 14 spent between $2,500 and slightly more than $5,000.

present annual contributions of another foundation to several carefully selected university schools are of pronounced value both in permitting the particular schools to concentrate greater attention on preparation of faculty for nursing education, and as a demonstration of the foundation's conviction of the social importance of the nurse. Gifts such as these need to be reproduced hundreds of times over, and with comparable discriminative judgment in the selection of recipients.

In Financing the Future of Higher Education, Dr. Thad Lewis Hungate has described trends, conspicuous since 1920, in the decreasing importance of philanthropic contributions to higher education, and the sharp decline in the proportion of gifts and bequests made for purposes of endowment.[1] Many small donors have replaced a few large donors and probably close to half of all contributions are now earmarked for current and general use.

Should these trends continue, the day may already have ended when schools of nursing can even hope for endowments such as those that have permitted much of the phenomenal development of medical education. However, it is believed that some such funds, particularly in the form of bequests, might still be obtained for endowment. If contributed in substantial amounts by many donors to schools prepared to benefit to the maximum, current expendable funds would permit those schools to develop areas of teaching and research that cannot now be cultivated. Were universities to reevaluate their expenditures, undesignated university funds might also be made available to a larger degree than at present. A very disturbing aspect of fiscal policy is the negligible amount that appears to be contributed from general university income to the operation of schools of nursing. For universities to allocate funds on the basis of pressure exerted by a few of their constituent units or by external forces that may be of transitory or secondary importance, only continues the neglect of a field of professional education concerned with the protection of life itself.

[1] New York, Teachers College, Columbia University, 1946, pp. 111–149.

That public as well as private support of nursing education is essential is a foregone conclusion. Just as higher education has been expanding more rapidly in public than in private institutions, so nursing education is likely to find proportionately greater opportunity within universities and colleges maintained by public support. Already a considerable number of state and municipal universities have introduced basic or advanced curricula or both, and several others are considering the advisability of taking this step.

Not since the end of World War I has there been such widespread reexamination of higher education as now. Studies by individual persons, educational institutions, and official bodies, including the President's Commission on Higher Education, evidence the interest in planning for sounder curricula and enlarged educational opportunities. Although it is assumed that private institutions will contribute to expansion to whatever degree possible, there is wide consensus that public universities and colleges will be required to bear major responsibility for any appreciable increase in enrollments and expensive new professional schools.

Many see in this reawakened interest an auspicious occasion for nursing education to make strong representation, especially to official bodies, concerning the necessity for larger financing and the establishment of more collegiate schools. The experience of nurses who have administered curricula in public institutions serves to strengthen this conclusion. These administrators generally testify that public universities are less bound to tradition than are their private counterparts and hence are more willing to experiment in uncultivated areas; that they are often more responsive to social pressures and social needs; and that the financial sources on which they draw are probably less precarious.

Should both private and public universities rapidly expand facilities for nursing education well beyond what is now available, there is grave fear that the achievement would still be inadequate.

169

Because professional education in nursing has to be built almost "from the ground up" in many parts of the country, supplementary federal assistance is viewed by a large proportion of informed nurses as necessary and desirable. Those who question the desirability do it chiefly through concern that federal funds would not be made available to private schools, which provide a large proportion of existing facilities for the preparation of nurses. Perhaps partly because nurse educators gained much confidence in the government from their participation during the war in the program of the United States Cadet Nurse Corps, relatively little anxiety is expressed about "federal control" of nursing education.

A major reason federal assistance is regarded as necessary is that sufficient numbers of collegiate nurse students cannot otherwise be obtained, it is believed, who are able to pay a considerable part of the cost of their education. The President's Commission on Higher Education reports that prior to World War II student tuition and other required fees produced approximately 19 per cent of the income of public and 60 per cent of the income of private colleges and universities.[1] By 1947 the percentages had risen to the alarming figures of roughly 35 and 78 respectively. Much of the income from fees in the latter year was paid, to be sure, by the government in behalf of those students entitled to G.I. benefits. Where students for nursing curricula, in other than small numbers, can be found when federal payments cease is not known, particularly since nursing has never yet drawn a proportionate share of its constituency from economically privileged families that are both accustomed and able to send their daughters to college.

Under such circumstances nurse educators examined with profound interest the Report of the President's Commission that recommended elimination of all student fees on the junior college

[1] Higher Education for American Democracy; A Report of the President's Commission on Higher Education. Washington, U. S. Government Printing Office, 1947, vol. 5, pp. 33–34.

level; rolling back of other fees to nearer the 1939 proportions; establishment of a broad national program of scholarships; and granting of federal assistance to institutions of higher learning for both day-to-day operations and capital outlay.

Even greater was the interest taken in the introduction in the Senate on April 30, 1948 of the bill, S. 2588, to provide grants and scholarships for medical, dental, nursing, and public health education. Recognition of the extreme shortage of personnel in the several health services motivated the drawing of this bill, intended to aid schools to meet costs of instruction, expansion of faculty and students, and construction of new buildings; and to induce greater numbers of young men and women, through provision of scholarships, to prepare to enter these services. Unfortunately no final action was taken on this bill before the Congress adjourned.

However, its clauses applicable to nursing are instructive as an indication of the amount and conditions of assistance under consideration. Grants to "both graduate and undergraduate" schools of nursing were set at $15,000,000 for the first fiscal year, $18,000,000 for the next year, and thereafter at such sums "as may be necessary." Provision was included to enable the Surgeon General of the United States Public Health Service to make grants "from time to time" to assist, up to 50 per cent of the cost, in the construction of buildings and other facilities in basic schools, "whether or not they are degree granting," and in advanced schools. Also provided was reimbursement through the Surgeon General to states for scholarships not to exceed 10 per cent of the students enrolled "for the standard course." A scholarship was defined as covering cost of tuition, educational fees, and books during the entire length "of the standard course."

Throughout the bill emphasis was placed on the fact that assistance should be provided only to schools that admitted students without discrimination as to race, creed, color, or national origin. In states where separate facilities are required by law to be maintained for "separate racial groups," grants could

171

be made to schools that "admit members of the minority racial groups," and to other schools provided "the Surgeon General finds that there are comparable opportunities for qualified members of such racial groups who reside in the State to obtain the type of professional training offered by such school."

Prior to the introduction of this proposed legislation a committee composed of the six major professional associations in nursing had formulated "essentials to be included in a bill providing for federal aid for nursing education." The Committee was strongly of the opinion that federal funds should be used primarily as an instrumentality for improving the quality of nursing education and nursing service. During the war emphasis had to be centered chiefly upon quantity. Hence hundreds of weak hospital schools operating apprenticeship forms of training had received financial aid. In order that effort might be redirected toward constructive long-range goals, the Committee concluded that federal appropriations should be used to provide: assistance for the improvement of basic and advanced nursing programs; aid in research and experimental work in nursing service and nursing education conducted under contract with appropriate professional nursing associations; assistance for temporary demonstrations, intensive courses, and workshops in nursing education; scholarships for qualified graduate nurses to enable them to further their preparation for a nursing specialty; and funds for the effective administration of the enabling act.

Although the Committee recognized the categories of both hospital schools and college and university schools, whether under public or private auspices, as eligible for federal assistance, it insisted that aid should be restricted to those schools that received approval as meeting certain established criteria. The Senate bill also stated that only schools, "which are approved or accredited by a body or bodies approved by the Surgeon General for such purposes, shall be considered." The Committee's "essentials," however, went much farther than did the Senate bill—or

172

any prospective legislation could perhaps wisely go—in defining methods for creation of criteria and granting of approval, and for the formulation of other important policies.

Here matters rest at present. All persons desirous of having federal aid made available to nursing education hope that legislation will be enacted in the next session of the Congress. Representatives of the six professional nursing associations will supposedly strive to have subsequent congressional bills more sharply drawn to emphasize the qualitative as well as the quantitative aspects of the problem to be solved.

We must now return to the question specifically under consideration in this section: the financing of college and university schools of nursing. Because of the great and immediate need for funds resulting from society's earlier failure to provide for this essential health service, *we recommend that individual persons, informed groups, and private corporate bodies including foundations and institutions of higher learning themselves, make the largest possible sums available for the creation or strengthening of soundly conceived college and university schools of nursing. We recommend, further, that official bodies—local, state, and federal—concern themselves at once with supplying whatever additional resources are necessary for the adequate support of nursing education on the professional, as well as the nonprofessional, level. We recommend, finally, that all contributions and grants be made, not on the basis of the auspices under which schools are operated, but rather on the basis of educational standards maintained by individual schools.*

VII

RESOURCES FOR THE FUTURE

PREVIOUSLY figures have been cited for the number of hospital schools of nursing that have established affiliations with institutions of higher learning, and of advanced curricula offered by universities and colleges. The more important consideration of the number of basic curricula operated by universities and colleges, however, has purposely been postponed until now when it might be examined within the larger context of resources needed for the future.

EXISTING COLLEGIATE SCHOOLS CONTRASTED WITH RESOURCES NEEDED

Of the 1,214 schools of nursing that supplied statistical data as of January 1, 1946 to the National League of Nursing Education, 77, or 6 per cent, reported that they were organized in and controlled by institutions of higher learning—47 were in universities and 30 in colleges. Of the total number 40 offered only a degree program; 29 offered both a degree and a diploma program; and 8 offered only a diploma. In justice to schools in the last two categories it should be recalled that some of the diploma programs were adaptations to the war situation and are now being ended. Figures for the number of degrees conferred in 1947 by 67 schools indicate that only 1,327 students, or an average of just under 20 per school, received either the bachelor's or the master's degree. Since only two university schools grant the master's degree upon completion of the basic curriculum, most of the degrees obviously were the baccalaureate.

174

Between January 1946 and January 1948, when the National League made its latest request for information about enrollments, three of the 77 schools had closed or were in the process of closing. This one fact gives some indication of the precariousness of the base on which schools of nursing may be operated within institutions of higher learning. One school failed to submit requested data. The total enrollment in the basic curriculum of the 73 reporting schools was 9,307 students, of whom 4,889, or 52.5 per cent, were registered in the degree program. In the 66 schools known to give such a program the size of the student body working for a degree ranged from 3 to 214, with a median of 67. Nineteen schools had enrollments between 100 and 200, and only one had more.

If we select from these data for recapitulation those that will most readily help us visualize existing resources in number of basic degree curricula and students enrolled, we note that there are now 66 schools conducting basic degree programs, with a total matriculation in them of fewer than 5,000 and a median of only 67. It is probable that well under 1,500 will receive a degree in 1948, of whom all except about 100 will receive the baccalaureate.

In contrast there are 70 degree-conferring medical schools, with a total enrollment in 1946–1947 of 23,471 students and a median of 295. The number of their graduates in that year was 6,389. To carry the comparison farther, it should be noted that 56 medical schools were within universities, 2 were operated by colleges, and 12 were independent. More than a third of the degree-conferring schools of nursing were controlled by colleges, most of which have nothing like the financial and educational resources of the 56 universities with medical schools that rank among the foremost institutions of higher learning in the United States. Of these universities 37 also operated basic schools of nursing, but 19 had never undertaken responsibility for a form of professional education that would seem of correlative social importance.

175

The question now arises of the resources that will be required for the future. Particularly for the sake of those persons who had hoped that specific figures could be given in this report for the number of each kind of educational undertaking needed—whether schools for practical nurses, bedside nurses, or professional nurses on both the basic and advanced levels—and also for the approximate number of students who should be trained in each kind of school, we regret that no such definite data are now possible. Those persons rightfully assumed that specific figures would be almost indispensable to planning for the long-range future of nursing. Comprehensive studies which would run into years of work and hundreds of thousands of dollars, however, are as yet lacking. It must also be taken into consideration that in a period when health services are undergoing such drastic changes, the very existence of stated estimates for ultimate goals might serve to freeze a situation that is now dynamic and should remain so, at least until more experimentation and experience are available regarding allocation of functions to persons with different kinds of preparation.

If it is not possible, however, to present the figures desired, the direction along which change should move appears clear. Suggestions have already been offered to the effect that schools for practical nurses should be developed during the next few years as rapidly as planning for sound establishment and wise distribution will permit; that several hundred socially undesirable hospital schools should be closed; that advanced curricula within universities and colleges should be restudied and greatly strengthened. The desirability of these changes is unmistakable. Equally unmistakable is the need for development and cultivation of basic schools of nursing in institutions of higher learning to go on apace.

The present number of basic degree schools is probably not large enough. What is more important, however, are the clinical, financial, and teaching resources at their disposal, and the num-

176

ber of students they can attract. Individually there is wide varia-
tion among them, but as a group the current 66 schools are not
satisfactory in any of these respects. Some are said to be so unsatisfactory that their continuation should be questioned.

The constituency of the Association of Collegiate Schools of
Nursing throws some light on this situation. The Association was
created in 1935 with 21 charter members "to develop nursing
education on a professional and collegiate level; to promote and
strengthen the relationships between nursing and institutions of
higher education; and to promote study and experimentation in
nursing service and nursing education." It has consistently maintained that its fundamental purpose was to bring together only
those institutions that are free to control and able to support
their educational policies. The development of sound standards
has been considered more important than size of membership. Its
requirements, examples of which have been cited under the discussion of faculty and financial structure, are so reasonable, however, that any school established on a base that educators generally consider sound would have little difficulty in securing
membership.

At present the Association has 34 active and 7 associate members. Of the former, 7 represent schools giving only the basic
curriculum, 12 giving both basic and advanced curricula, and 15
only advanced curricula. Of the associate members, 5 offer only
the basic course of study, and 2 offer both. Hence a mere 26, out
of 66 schools now providing basic work leading to the degree,
have received the recognition of this body. How many more
might be able to qualify is not known, but it can be safely
assumed that the number is not large.

Under such circumstances the task of the future is decisive. It is
to strengthen further schools that hold or are eligible for membership in the Association of Collegiate Schools of Nursing; to recon-
sider whether schools that are unlikely to be able to meet some
such reasonable standards within the next few years should con-

tinue; and to establish new professional schools where surveys indicate they are most needed, would receive substantial financial support, and would attract sufficiently large student bodies. As a goal toward which to work during the next decade, *we recommend that effort be directed to building basic schools of nursing in universities and colleges, comparable in number to existing medical schools, that are sound in organizational and financial structure, adequate in facilities and faculty, and well distributed to serve the needs of the entire country.*

In the light of the present dearth of professional nurses and of the functions that have been outlined as requiring their services, some 70 collegiate schools of nursing with a student body of 20,000 might prove too small to meet the demand. If so, the fact would become apparent with time. At present the need is for concentration of attention upon a goal that is attainable and that could serve as a sound foundation for any further developments.

Desirability of Broad Planning

One of the major reasons for the present weakness of many collegiate schools of nursing is the almost fortuitous way in which they have been established. Representatives of hospital schools who have seen the growing trend toward administration of professional education by institutions of higher learning have convinced colleges and universities of the desirability of operating schools of nursing. Arrangements have often been made without adequate consideration of the extensiveness of clinical facilities, faculty, and financing essential to maintain a professional school, and without giving thought to its contribution beyond serving local needs.

Although the lack of wisdom of such impromptu action should long since have become apparent, individual hospital schools continue to strive either to establish affiliation with, or to come under the aegis of, institutions of higher education. What is particularly hazardous is their inclination to carry on negotiations with universities or colleges before consulting responsible groups that might be interested in planning for the future of nursing education at least on a statewide basis. If this process continues, the country will be burdened with a large number of weak, badly located collegiate schools that contribute little in prestige or usefulness either to themselves or to nursing education generally. Faced by the tragic example of where proliferation of hospital schools has led the profession, one might assume that nurse educators would avoid any drift in the same direction by collegiate schools.

If this current tendency is to be offset and professional nursing education is to be put on a sounder foundation, systematic and objective planning on a broad base is requisite. Mention has already been made of the fact that some officially appointed state commissions, authorized to examine hospital and perhaps other health needs, have asked that surveys be made of requisite nursing personnel and facilities for its preparation. At least in principle these undertakings are so encouraging that we believe nursing should initiate requests for inclusion of such surveys where official groups have overlooked their importance.

A state office of higher education, or state commission created to plan for expansion of educational facilities, is another body that might appropriately be asked to concern itself with the determination of need for collegiate schools of nursing. Not long ago the legislature of a jurisdiction that had never operated a state university authorized the appointment of a temporary commission charged with formulating recommendations for the establishment of such an institution. Prior to preparing its report, an examination was made of existing facilities for several kinds of professional education, including nursing. Although this state is more fortunate than most in the number of nursing students enrolled in degree-conferring institutions, it was recommended that because of the shortage of nurse teachers, supervisors, and

179

administrators, schools be created within two proposed medical centers designed to offer preparation for several health services. It was also suggested that practical nurses might advantageously be trained under the auspices of junior colleges, which were advocated as part of the state system of higher education.

Wherever a statewide body is engaged in the development of either health services or higher education, nurses should attempt if possible to work within it. Thus their task of interpretation of need to the public might be greatly lessened, and they might find a more substantial place for professional education through cooperative rather than separate effort. In many jurisdictions, however, any broad planning for nursing education will unquestionably have to be initiated and pursued in early stages by the profession itself. In a few states committees, generally sponsored by the state League of Nursing Education but in at least one jurisdiction by a council composed of all the nursing associations, are engaged in the task of attempting to evaluate needs and plan for requisite kinds and amounts of nursing education.

The chief fear about these committees is the likelihood that they will assume that planning for the future is possible on the basis of such facts and opinions as can be supplied at the conference table, and that the resulting blueprint can then be transformed into operating programs without broad community participation. Whether representatives of the health services and of education should be brought into the planning process immediately after its initiation or somewhat later cannot be categorically stated. It is difficult, however, to visualize sound constructive action without their continuing assistance and cooperation. Almost certainly research will need to be an essential part of the process. No group of persons, however well informed about nursing education in the particular state, has enough basic data for construction of a blueprint. After the design has been completed, a carefully prepared program of public education, devised to lead to public participation and support, is almost a necessity.[1]

Planning and subsequent action on anything more than a local basis are large undertakings that require time, patience, careful thought, experienced personnel, and money. So important, however, are they and so great is the current interest in nursing that it is believed support can be found for the drawing of a blueprint. It is also believed that representatives of newspapers, radio, and the public platform, as well as members of the health services and education, will willingly contribute their services to a program of public information.

Committees should be concerned with all types of preparation for nursing. Although their particular interest may lie in degree-conferring schools of nursing, nothing short of consideration of need for each kind of training, including that for practical and graduate bedside nurses, will provide the guidance essential, or afford perspective even for seeing in what amount collegiate preparation should be supplied.

Although the discussion has thus far emphasized statewide planning, it must not be concluded that the state is necessarily the best geographical unit for purposes of planning. Because government and professional associations are thus set up, action is often facilitated thereby. In many instances, however, regional planning might offer more fruitful results, and in some respects national planning is important. As categories of training become more complex and expensive and the schools providing them fewer in number, the geographical area under review should become progressively larger.

To illustrate, in-service training is generally thought to be the exclusive concern of the particular institution or corporation. Since it is an instrumentality for increasing the efficiency of all personnel employed, an institution should clearly have an inter-

---

[1] Of distinct value as a guide for broad planning of nursing education are the principles of community organization discussed by Dr. Leonard W. Mayo in his paper, "Community Planning for Nursing Care," presented on June 3, 1948 to the Biennial Nursing Convention in Chicago.

est in utilizing it. The obligation of the nursing profession and the public does not extend beyond indicating to directors of nursing service its signal achievements in industry; its potentialities for quickly making untrained personnel competent to handle, under supervision, situations requiring considerable technical skill; and its value in giving trained personnel knowledge of new facts, theories, and procedures. But the obligation of the nursing profession and the public regarding preparation of practical and graduate bedside nurses is different. If the training of these two groups purports to be of an educational nature, rather than in-service provided solely to enhance hospital efficiency, it is charged with a public interest and should be subject to public regulation, including determination of its distribution. Because relatively numerous and simple units to supply these types of preparation are required, planning for statewide distribution should be adequate.

This generalization is not equally true when professional preparation is considered. Some collegiate schools may be expected to serve state needs primarily; others should be conceived to serve the needs of a region; a few to serve more than one region or the nation at large.

The part of the United States known to experts in regionalism as the Southeast has recently given much thought to regional education. The fact that the issue of separate educational facilities for Negro and white students has been brought into the discussion of plans for the future, should not blind persons interested in education to the positive aspects of this thinking. The several states of the Southeast concluded that they could not individually afford to maintain advanced graduate work in various fields, laboratories and libraries for advanced research, and the more expensive or numerically less needed professional schools. They concluded that by pooling their resources such advanced preparation could be supplied on a high level of attainment. An official council has already been created. It has